Take Charge of Your

HEALTH

Take Charge of Your
HEALTH

Exercising and Eating Right Are Your Best Defenses for
Preventing Chronic Diseases and Being in Great Shape!

SUZANNE O'BRIEN

Personal Fitness Trainer

To order additional copies of this book, contact:
Xlibris Corporation
1-888-795-4274
www.Xlibris.com
Orders@Xlibris.com
44430

Contents

Introduction 9

What Is Diabetes? 11

Who Gets Diabetes? 16

The Diabetic Difference 22

Oral Hypoglycemics 31

What Is Osteoporosis? 32

How Is Osteoporosis Diagnosed? 34

Exercises That Prevent Osteoporosis 36

Hormone-Replacement Therapy 42

Medications Approved for Increasing Bone Mass 43

What Is Heart Disease? 44

High Blood Pressure 45

Long-Term Complications of High Blood Pressure 49

Medicines That Treat High Blood Pressure 51

Preventing High Blood Pressure 52

Coronary Artery Disease 54

Preventing Coronary Artery Disease 56

Let's Get Moving! 57

Cardiorespiratory Fitness 63

Muscular Strength and Endurance 69

Types of Weight Training Exercises 73

The Weight Training Exercises 77

A Few Simple Stretches 90

Your Upper Body Workout 93

Your Lower Body Workouts and Exercises 103

Flexibility 119

Assessing Flexibility 122

Flexibility Exercises 124

Nutrition 137

Proteins 138

Fats 139

Carbohydrates 142

Fiber 144

Vitamins 146

Minerals 147

Amazing Antioxidants 149

Fantastic Phytochemicals 150

Your Thirty-Day Fitness Program 151

To my son, Nicholas.

With Love Always,
Mom

Introduction

At the present time, health care in America has reached an all time low. If you are lucky enough to have insurance, there is so much red tape involved to get the treatment you need, and doctors are so overworked that it may take weeks or months to get an appointment with them. When you are lucky enough to see one, the visit can be so rushed that you go away feeling like you went on a roller-coaster ride that stopped abruptly and left you confused and unsure of what was actually accomplished. Welcome to health care today.

As a registered nurse, I have seen the devastation that disease can do to a person's life. I have also seen the treatment programs and their outcomes for countless patients.

I will tell you this—it is possible to "manage" some chronic diseases, and the level of management depends on two factors: One, the education the patient is given about the disease and what is needed to successfully manage it; two, the expertise of the doctor himself.

There are new advances being made in the treatment and care of chronic diseases every day, so it is very important to make sure that the doctor you choose is up-to-date on the latest information. Unfortunately, doctors are not gods, and controlling chronic conditions can be hit-or-miss. The medications used to treat these conditions have some terrible side effects.

Okay, so you're thinking this is depressing. Is this what I have to look forward to in my future? The good news is that, by reading this book and educating yourself, you can prevent the most common debilitating diseases affecting tens of millions of people today. With moderate adjustments in lifestyle (exercise and diet), you can prevent the development of chronic illness and, at the same time, you will look and feel better than you ever have! How's that for good news!

There are three chronic conditions that can have devastating effects on people when they are left untreated. They are diabetes, osteoporosis, and heart disease. In the following chapters, you will learn what these diseases are, how a person gets them, and most importantly, how to prevent them!

What Is Diabetes?

Diabetes is a chronic disease that cannot be cured, but can be controlled with education and effort. Diabetes is a metabolic disorder resulting from an inability of the body to break down sugar (glucose) properly. When a person eats food, the stomach produces chemicals that break down the food particles into small substances that travel through the intestines; the body keeps the nutrients it can use and sends those molecules into the bloodstream where they are carried to places in the body that need them. The material it does not need is excreted out of the body as waste. When we consume food, there are three categories of nutrients that we eat: protein, carbohydrates, and fats. Diabetes is caused by an inability of the body to process carbohydrates.

Carbohydrates are broken down by the body into glucose, which is another name for sugar. When we eat, the amount of glucose in our bloodstream temporarily rises until it is absorbed to provide fuel. When a person has diabetes, glucose cannot be adequately absorbed by the cells; and as a result, sugar levels rise. This increase of glucose in the blood damages the body. Excessive sugar levels, called high blood sugar, are a continuing health risk for every person with diabetes and must be controlled.

Insulin—The Helper Hormone

As we said before, after we eat, glucose levels in the blood rise. Within about ten minutes, insulin, a hormone produced by the pancreas, aids glucose to be taken into individual cells and stores it there for use in the future. Insulin is produced by a gland called the pancreas located just behind and below the stomach. There is a group of cells hanging off the pancreas called the islets of Langerhans. These islet cells are where insulin is secreted. If you have diabetes, you have a problem with insulin. Either your pancreas does not secrete any insulin (as in type I diabetes) or you have insulin resistance (as in type II diabetes). In the case of insulin resistance, your pancreas secretes insulin, usually in excessive amounts; but the insulin receptor sites at the cells no longer work properly, and insulin is unable to bind at the cell. In this situation, glucose is unable to be used for fuel and stays floating in the bloodstream.

As I just mentioned, there are two main types of diabetes. Type I, also known as insulin-dependent diabetes mellitus and type II, also known as noninsulin-dependent diabetes mellitus.

Type I Diabetes (IDDM)

Only about 10 percent of people with diabetes have type I. Type I used to be called juvenile-onset because most of the time people developed it in childhood. But the name has changed because a small percentage is being diagnosed with it later in life. With type I diabetes, the pancreas produces no insulin at all, and the treatment is insulin injections. Doctors believe that the cause of type I diabetes is an autoimmune response, which means that the body actually attacks and destroys part of itself. This response is usually triggered by a virus. When the body has an infection, it produces antibodies to fight the bacteria that cause the infection. But in the case of type I diabetes, the body makes antibodies that destroy its own tissue. An enzyme in the pancreas that seems to be the target of this autoimmune attack has been identified. Researchers have been able to use a blood test based on this enzyme to identify people who are at risk for developing type I diabetes.

Symptoms of Type I Diabetes (IDDM)

1. Weight Loss—You lose weight as your body loses glucose in the urine, and your body breaks down muscle and fat to use for energy.
2. Frequent Urination—When your blood glucose is greater than 180 mg/dl, your kidneys can't filter it back into the bloodstream, and it spills out into your urine. The large amount of glucose in your urine makes the urine so concentrated that water is drawn out of the blood and into the urine to reduce the concentration of glucose in the urine. This water and glucose continuously fill up the bladder and cause frequent urination.
3. Increase in Thirst—Your thirst increases because you are losing so much water in your urine and your body has become dehydrated.
4. Increased Hunger—Your cells are hungry because they cannot get the glucose they need, and as a result, you feel hungry all the time.
5. Weakness—Your body feels weak because you are not able to utilize fuel for energy.

Normal blood glucose is steadily kept between 60 and 115 mg/dl. In type I diabetes, blood sugars can reach life-threatening high levels as much as 400-600 mg/dl. This is due to the absolute lack of insulin production. High blood sugar is also known as hyperglycemia. ""Hyper" means high; "glycemia" means sugar.".

Diabetic Ketoacidosis—The most severe complication of type I diabetes is diabetic ketoacidosis. When the body is unable to use any glucose for fuel, it starts to break down fat for energy. As fat is broken down, ketone bodies are produced and begin to accumulate in the blood and spill into the urine. Ketone bodies are acidic and lead to nausea, abdominal pain, and sometimes vomiting. The large amount of water leaving the body with the glucose causes important electrolytes such as sodium and potassium to be depleted. All these abnormalities can cause a person to become very drowsy and possibly lose consciousness. This is a life-threatening condition and must be identified and corrected quickly or death can result.

Type II Diabetes (NIDDM)

Type II diabetes used to be called maturity-onset or adult-onset diabetes because most people developed it after age forty. Type II is also called noninsulin-dependent diabetes mellitus or NIDDM. This is because most people with this type of diabetes do not need to take insulin. Approximately, 18 million people in the United States have type II diabetes, and a third or more have it but do not know it. In type II diabetes, the pancreas continues to function, but either too little insulin is produced or the insulin that is produced is used ineffectively due to insulin resistance right at the cells. Eighty percent of the people with type II diabetes are overweight. Fat cells are insulin resistant and may prevent the body from using insulin effectively. Being overweight is the number one risk factor in getting type II diabetes. Even a person who is only moderately overweight increases his risk. Studies show that being only 20 percent more than the desirable weight doubles the chance of getting diabetes.

Many people with type II diabetes make more than enough insulin, but the insulin they make cannot be utilized due to insulin resistance at the cell. It is believed that overeating, especially the wrong foods, has worn out the insulin receptor sites and insulin can no longer bind to these sites. The result is glucose cannot be taken into the cells to be used as fuel.

Symptoms of Type II Diabetes (NIDDM)

1. Frequent Urination and Thirst—You are urinating more frequently than usual, which dehydrates your body and leaves you thirsty.
2. Fatigue—Your body is unable to get the energy it needs to carry on the activities of daily living.
3. Slow Healing of Infections—Your white blood cells, which help with healing and defending against infections, don't perform correctly in the high-glucose environment present in your body when you have diabetes. The organisms that cause infections can survive and multiply at a much greater rate in a high-glucose environment. If you have diabetes, you are more susceptible to infections.

4. Genital Itching—Yeast infections also love a high-glucose environment. So diabetes in females usually brings about the itching and discomfort of yeast infections.

5. Numbness in the Feet or Legs—Neuropathy is a long-term complication from diabetes. If you have numbness, you have probably had diabetes for a long time because neuropathy takes more than five years to develop in a person with diabetes.

6. Obesity—If you are obese, you are much more likely to develop diabetes than if you maintained an ideal weight, but being obese alone does not mean you have diabetes.

7. Blood Glucose—Normal blood glucose is between 60 and 115 mg/dl in people. With type II diabetes, blood glucose levels are usually somewhere around 200 to 250 mg/dl.

Type II diabetes has a strong heredity factor. This means that if someone in your family such as parents or grandparents has the disease, you are more likely to get it than if none of your relatives has it. The great news is that the risk factors associated with type II diabetes are preventable. So with some changes in lifestyle (eating healthy food and exercising), you can avoid acquiring the disease. If you already have it, these same adjustments can help control your blood sugar so that complications due to high blood sugar will never affect you.

Gestational Diabetes

There is another form of diabetes that I need to mention even though it occurs only in 2 percent of all pregnancies.

During pregnancy, the growing fetus and the placenta create various hormones to help the fetus grow. Some of these hormones have other characteristics such as anti-insulin properties that decrease your body's sensitivity to insulin, increase glucose production, and therefore, cause gestational diabetes during pregnancy.

At about the twentieth week of pregnancy, your body produces enough of these hormones to block your insulin's normal actions and cause diabetes. After your baby is born, the fetus and placenta are no longer in your body; so their anti-insulin hormones are gone, and your gestational diabetes disappears.

It is important to note that even though diabetes subsides after you give birth, type II diabetes develops within fifteen years after the pregnancy in more than half of the women who had gestational diabetes. This high number is probably the result from a genetic susceptibility to diabetes in these women that is intensified by the large amount of anti-insulin hormones in their bodies during pregnancy.

A woman who is pregnant should be tested for gestational diabetes around the twenty-fourth to twenty-eighth week of her pregnancy.

How Is Diabetes Diagnosed?

As mentioned earlier, the most common symptoms of diabetes are:

1. frequent urination and thirst,
2. fatigue,
3. weight loss (most common in type I),
4. slow-healing infections.

The definition of diabetes mellitus is excessive glucose in the blood. The American Diabetes Association published new updated standards for the positive diagnosis of diabetes, which includes any one of the following three criteria:

1. *Blood Glucose*—of greater than or equal to 200 mg/dl when tested two hours (2HPG) after ingesting seventy-five grams of glucose by mouth. This test is called the oral glucose tolerance test. This test is known as the standard for the diagnosis of diabetes.
2. *Casual Plasma Glucose*—concentration greater than or equal to 200 mg/dl along with symptoms of diabetes.
3. *Fasting Plasma Glucose* (FPG)—of greater than or equal to 126 mg/dl. Fasting means that the person has not eaten any food eight hours prior to the test. You may also have a blood glucose level that is not a positive diagnosis for diabetes but shows that a person has impaired glucose tolerance.

   - FPG less than 110 mg/dl is a normal fasting glucose.
   - FPG greater than or equal to 110 mg/dl but less than 126 mg/dl is considered impaired fasting glucose.
   - FPG equal to or greater than 126 mg/dl on more than one occasion is a definitive diagnosis of diabetes.
   - 2HPG less than 140 mg/dl is normal glucose tolerance.
   - 2HPG greater than or equal to 140 mg/dl but less than 200 mg/dl is impaired glucose tolerance.
   - 2HPG equal to or greater than 200 mg/dl on more than one occasion gives a positive diagnosis of diabetes.

Who Gets Diabetes?

Who Gets Type I Diabetes?

We said before that type I diabetes is an autoimmune disease, which means that your body attacks and destroys a part of itself. In the case of type I diabetes, the body destroys the insulin-producing beta cells of the pancreas. There are identifiable risk factors in getting type I diabetes, including genetics and ethnicity. For example, if your parents or grandparents have type I diabetes, you are more likely to develop it. Caucasians are also at higher risk of getting type I diabetes than Hispanics or African Americans. Doctors have been able to identify a protein in the blood called islet cell antibodies found in people who a few years later develop the disease. There is also an abnormal chromosome found on the DNA of people who are predisposed to getting type I diabetes.

Even though a doctor can identify a person who is predisposed to getting type I diabetes, there must be an outside factor that triggers the disease. Experts believe that there are several different viruses that trigger this autoimmune response, and one of the viruses could be the common cold.

Who Gets Type II Diabetes?

Researchers estimate that by the year 2020, about 250 million people worldwide may be at significant risk for developing type II diabetes.

There are risk factors a person can change and risk factors that cannot be changed. Those that cannot be changed are age—most cases of type II diabetes occur in people over age forty-five; ethnicity—insulin resistance, which is a major cause of type II diabetes seems to have a higher incidence (twice as high) among blacks and Hispanics and even higher among Native Americans; previous diagnosis of gestational diabetes—a woman who has had gestational diabetes during one or more of her pregnancies has a 50 percent chance of developing type II diabetes later in life; genetics—much more common finding in people with type II diabetes, but environmental factors such as obesity and lack of exercise trigger the disease.

Identifiable Risk Factors that Can Be Changed

Obesity—Obesity is the number one risk factor for acquiring type II diabetes. Excessive fat, especially fat around the belly, is insulin resistant. This resistance is a major trigger for type II diabetes. Even losing 5-10 percent of your weight can dramatically reduce your chance of getting diabetes.

Physical Inactivity—Physical inactivity has a high association with diabetes. When you are active, your body burns more sugar for energy. Researchers have also found that exercise increases the individual cell's sensitivity to insulin, thus decreasing the incidence of insulin resistance.

What Are the Complications of Diabetes?

There are several short-term and long-term complications of diabetes. Short-term Complications—Short-term complications are those situations that come about rapidly and can be resolved quickly as well. The most common type of short-term complication is *hypoglycemia.* "Hypo"—low; "glycemia"—sugar. Hypoglycemia is most often caused as a result to treating your high blood sugar. Your doctor prescribes insulin or oral hypoglycemic drugs in an effort to keep your blood sugar as close to normal as possible. If you exercise too much, don't have enough to eat or take too much medication, your blood glucose can drop to a level at which symptoms appear. Your brain and body need a constant supply of glucose at all times to function properly. Your brain needs glucose to think clearly, and your muscles need glucose to do physical work. When your blood glucose drops to 60 mg/dl or below, you will start to experience the following symptoms:

1. Pale skin color
2. Feeling of hunger
3. Sweating
4. Rapid heart beat
5. Anxiety
6. Headache
7. Loss of concentration
8. Visual disturbances
9. Confusion
10. Convulsions
11. Coma, unconsciousness

Hyperglycemia—Hyperglycemia occurs when blood sugar levels are too high. The symptoms of hyperglycemia are increased thirst, frequent urination, fatigue, and unexplained weight loss. These symptoms are usually indications for a positive diagnosis of diabetes, but if your sugar is not being controlled properly, you may experience them after a diagnosis of diabetes has already been made.

Ketoacidosis—Ketoacidosis is a life-threatening short-term condition that affects only type I diabetics. The body starts to break down muscle and fat in order to make glucose. The end product of fat metabolism is ketone bodies. Ketones are acidic, and when high levels are in the bloodstream, the patient is said to be in ketoacidosis and must receive medical treatment immediately.

Symptoms of Ketoacidosis:

- Rapid Breathing—You experience rapid breathing when your blood is acidic and your body tries to blow off some of the acid through your lungs. Your breath has a fruity smell due to acetone.
- Nausea and Vomiting—You experience nausea and vomiting due to the buildup of acids and the loss of important electrolytes in the body.
- Drowsiness—Your blood is concentrated with glucose, but your brain is unable to use it.
- Weakness—You become weak because your muscles are unable to get the fuel they need.
- dehydration—Increased thirst and dry skin and tongue due to high glucose levels and the loss of water in the urine.
- The Hyperosmolar Syndrome—The hyperosmolar syndrome is similar to ketoacidosis in the fact that it creates ketones in your blood, but it doesn't make your blood acidic. Hyperosmolar syndrome usually affects the elderly with type II diabetes. It is brought on by the loss of large quantities of fluids through vomiting and diarrhea. This condition can develop over many days or weeks, and rapid breathing is not one of the symptoms due to the blood not becoming acidic.

Symptoms of Hyperosmolar Syndrome:

1. Frequent urination
2. Thirst
3. Weakness
4. Sunken eyeballs and rapid pulse due to dehydration
5. Decreased awareness/coma
6. Blood glucose of 600 mg/dl or higher

Hyperosmolar syndrome is life threatening and must be given medical attention immediately.

Long-Term Complications of Diabetes

Long-term complications are the most devastating effect of diabetes. Most long-term complications develop after ten years of having the disease. Many times in the case of type II diabetes, the first clue that the patient has the disease is the signs and symptoms of a long-term complication.

Doctors believe that years of high blood glucose levels adversely affect several parts of the body, leaving irreversible damage.

Kidney Disease

Your kidneys are the filtering system for your entire body. They get rid of harmful chemicals and other materials during the process of normal metabolism. Blood filters through the kidneys, trapping waste and sending it out in your urine. Nutrients the body can use are sent back into the bloodstream. The kidneys are also responsible for keeping a constant balance of water and salt in your body at all times.

At least 40 million Americans either have kidney disease or are at high risk for it, and many of them are diabetics.

When blood sugar levels are high, the kidneys have an increase in stress and pressure put on them because they are trying to rid the body of the extra glucose. This extra pressure overtime thickens the membranes in the kidneys, so they are unable to filter as much blood. If this situation continues for fifteen to twenty years without control of the high blood sugar, your kidneys may shut down entirely, and artificial means of cleansing your blood is necessary.

For ten to fifteen years, there are no obvious signs that the kidneys are failing, but your doctor can test for protein in the urine (which is an early sign of kidney disease). Normally, proteins are filtered back into the blood for future use, or a blood test can detect elevations in waste products in the blood—the blood urea nitrogen or BUN and the creatinine.

Your best defense against diabetic kidney disease is to control your blood sugar and keep it as close to normal as possible. This has been shown to avoid the onset of the disease and slow it down once it starts.

Eye Disease

Almost everyone who has diabetes shows some signs of an eye disease called retinopathy. Each year, as many as twenty-four thousand of diabetes patients lose their eyesight to the disease. High blood glucose affects all parts of the circulatory system, including the blood vessels of the eyes. The weakened capillaries (tiny blood vessels) of the eyes can leak and even rupture, releasing blood to form retinal hemorrhages. Hard exudates are formed as a result of the hemorrhages, and if they reach the macular area of the eye, vision is reduced or even lost.

A study involving more than 1,600 people with type I diabetes found that 67 percent developed retinopathy within five years of their diabetes diagnosis.

Keeping your blood sugar as close to normal as possible will prevent pressure on the blood vessels of the eyes. It is very important for the patient to have an eye exam by an ophthalmologist yearly to catch any early signs of eye damage.

Diabetic Neuropathy (Nerve Damage)

It is thought that nerve damage occurs due to a cutoff of blood to the nerve as a result of chemical toxins produced by the metabolism of too much glucose. Nerve damage results in the loss of sensation. Long nerves are the most commonly affected, and the feet usually suffer the most. Because high blood sugar causes slow healing of infections, a sore in the foot could lead to eventual amputation. An estimated six in one thousand people lose a limb to amputation.

To prevent neuropathic foot complications, it is vital that a person do a daily inspection of their feet. Check for any discoloration, swelling, or cuts. You can either use a large mirror or ask someone to look at the parts of your feet that you cannot see. Also, feel your feet. If one feels hot, it could be a sign of infection. Nerves are located throughout the body, and even though feet are the most susceptible, other parts of the body may be affected.

Loss of Bladder Fullness. You have nerves in your bladder that tell your brain that it is time to empty it. When you lose this sensation, urine is not eliminated, and urinary tract infections may result. You may also experience dribbling as a result of bladder fullness.

Constipation. The nerves of the intestines automatically contract and get rid of waste the body does not need. If the nerves of the intestines are not functioning properly, constipation will occur.

Gallbladder. The gallbladder is an organ that releases a substance called bile to help break down fat after a meal. If the gallbladder is not emptying properly, hard substances called gallstones may form.

Sexual Dysfunction. Fifty percent of males and 30 percent of females are affected. Males may not be able to sustain an erection, and females have trouble producing vaginal secretions for intercourse.

The good news about diabetic neuropathy is that when elevated blood glucose is brought down to normal, the symptoms improve and, in some cases, disappear.

Heart Disease

Coronary artery disease is the most common reason for death in type II patients. Type I patients are also at great risk. Coronary artery disease is the term for the progressive closure of the arteries, which supply blood to the heart muscle. When one or more of your arteries close, the result is a heart attack. High levels of glucose in the blood allow for fat and other substances to stick to the walls of the arteries. Overtime, they become more narrow and eventually shut.

There are several other risk factors that contribute to coronary artery disease:

Obesity. Being overweight puts increased stress on the heart.

Sedentary Lifestyle. When you are active, blood moves through your body more efficiently, and new blood vessels are made if there is an area that starts to become narrow.

Abnormal Levels of Triglycerides. Triglycerides are fats, and there are two types: LDL, or low-density lipoprotein, and HDL, or high-density lipoprotein. Your total triglyceride count should be less than 200 with LDL below 100 and HDL above 47. A high LDL count means that an increased number of fat particles are circulating in your blood and causing deposits on artery walls causing blockage.

All treatments of complications involve the control of blood sugar levels. Exercise and nutrition are also a major factor in decreasing a person's chance of getting coronary artery disease. We will discuss basic principles of fitness later in the book.

Gum Disease

Gum disease is often found in the diabetic patient due to the high concentration of glucose in the mouth. This promotes the growth of germs, which mix with food and saliva to form plaques on your gums.

To avoid getting gum disease, a person must first control blood sugar and brush their teeth at least twice a day and floss at least once a day.

The Diabetic Difference

Preventing diabetes and preventing the complications of diabetes are very similar. This is not applicable to preventing type I diabetes because it is triggered by an autoimmune response, but you can prevent type II, which is 90 percent of all diabetes cases.

You have two magic bullets when it comes to preventing diabetes. They are diet and exercise.

Exercise

Regular physical exercise is considered to be some form of activity done at least thirty minutes a day, three to five times a week. This could be walking, riding a bike, jogging, lifting weights, or any activity that will raise your heart rate or work your muscles.

The results of one study showed that when researchers assigned forty-one men with type II diabetes to a weight reduction and exercise program, after six years, half of the men no longer experienced diabetes symptoms.

Another study showed that 181 men with borderline diabetes who followed a similar program to lose weight and shape up showed normal blood sugar levels after five years.

Exercise requires a lot of energy. This means that your muscles must pull glucose from your bloodstream to feed cells. In addition, for up to two hours after you finish your workout, your muscles are busy clearing glucose out of your blood. Physical activity has been proven to increase the sensitivity of cells to insulin. This decreases the chance of insulin resistance, which is a major cause of getting type II diabetes.

Being overweight is the number one risk factor for acquiring type II diabetes, and regular physical activity will help you to lose those extra pounds. So whether you are trying to prevent getting diabetes or have the disease and want to control it, exercise is going to be a major part of your treatment plan. Later in this book, we will cover different types of exercises you can do; and you will be on your way to a healthier, happier, and fitter you!

Nutrition

As many as two-thirds of people with type II diabetes can manage the disease through diet and exercise alone.

What you eat is the cornerstone for preventing type II diabetes, and if you have diabetes, what you eat can help keep blood sugar at normal levels.

Being overweight is the number one risk factor for getting type II diabetes. Every time you eat, your pancreas shoots out insulin to lower the sugar in your blood. If you are eating in excess, your pancreas is being overworked as well and will eventually start to become unreactive. Fat cells are insulin resistant. If you have more body mass than is healthy, the insulin your body is producing will start to be unusable.

There are three classifications of nutrients that we eat: carbohydrates, proteins, and fat.

Carbohydrates break down into glucose and are the main source of energy for our bodies. Some common sources of carbohydrates are bread, potatoes, grains, cereals, and rice. There are two classifications of carbohydrates—refined and unrefined. You can think of refined carbohydrates to mean that a food item has been "processed." This means that it has been changed from its original form. Examples of refined carbohydrates are white bread, white sugar, candy, pasta, instant potatoes, and all packaged foods. When food is processed, many vitamins and minerals are taken out, and the beneficial nutrients are no longer there. As Grandpa used to say, "The whiter the bread, the quicker you're dead." Fruits, vegetables, and whole grains are also in the carbohydrate family; but they have not been processed and contain nutrients and fiber that are vital to good health. The sugar that is found in fruits is called fructose, and this sugar is absorbed slowly in the body, and blood sugar does not rise markedly as a result of eating it. It is probably due to excess carbohydrate consumption (refined ones) that most people are overweight. When the body has enough glucose in their cells to use as energy later on, excess glucose (carbohydrates) can be turned into fat and stored. Therefore, it is now recommended to eat a diet low in carbohydrates that are refined in order to maintain a desirable weight and healthy blood sugars.

Fiber

A very important component of unrefined carbohydrates is fiber. Fiber is not digestible and does not count as calories. Fiber also causes glucose to metabolize slower thus causing blood sugar to increase at a slower rate. Fiber is found in most fruits, grains, and vegetables. Fiber comes in two forms:

Soluble Fiber. This form of fiber dissolves in water and has been found to lower cholesterol and blood glucose.

Insoluble Fiber. This form of fiber cannot be dissolved in water. It absorbs water and stimulates movement in the intestines. Insoluble fiber prevents constipation and possibly colon cancer.

Fat

It has been stated that a person should have no more than 30 percent of his daily intake in fat. There are two types of fat, saturated fat and unsaturated fat.

Saturated Fat. This is the fat that comes from animal products. It is responsible for increasing cholesterol levels, which is responsible for the development of coronary artery disease, cerebrovascular disease, and peripheral vascular disease. The recommendation is no more than three hundred milligrams a day of fat from cholesterol.

Unsaturated Fat. This is the fat that comes from vegetable sources like canola oil and olive oil. This fat is the better choice. There are two classifications of unsaturated fat. They are monounsaturated fat and polyunsaturated fat. Even though the word "fat" has a negative connotation, your body requires what is known as essential fatty acids to function at its optimum level. The two most important types of fat you can eat are the polyunsaturates omega-3 and omega-6. The omega fats are found in cold-water fish such as salmon, tuna, cod, and their oils. They are also found in flax seed, walnuts, soybeans, wheat germs, sprouts, sea vegetables, and leafy greens. Omegas help raise your metabolism, help flush water from your kidneys, and lower your triglyceride levels.

"Good fat" is essential for health. It carries fat-soluble vitamins A, D, E, and K through the bloodstream. It:

— helps your body conserve protein;
— slows the absorption of carbohydrates to balance blood sugar levels;
— is a building block for production of estrogen, testosterone, and other hormones.

Protein

Protein is a source of nutrition that comes mostly from animals and their products such as milk and cheese. Protein contains no carbohydrates and does not raise blood glucose significantly. Animal products can have a very high fat content, so it is important to choose your meats carefully. Fish is also an excellent choice of protein with little or no fat in it. It is suggested that your diet contains 30 percent of protein daily.

Maintaining a healthy weight is vital to prevent type II diabetes and maintain healthy blood glucose levels if you have the disease. Later in the book, you will find a weight loss program that is easy to follow and will have you feeling great.

Eating a Balanced Diet

It is very important to get into the habit of eating a balanced diet with the appropriate carbohydrates. Different kinds of carbohydrates, because of their varying structure, are absorbed by the body in different ways. In the early 1980s, researchers developed a numeric system to measure the effects of carbohydrate-containing foods and blood sugar levels. The glycemic index (GI) ranks carbohydrates by how quickly they raise blood sugar within two to three hours of a meal. The numbers range from one to one hundred, with one hundred as the marker for pure glucose. The higher the number assigned to a food, the faster that food breaks down and raises blood sugar. Anything with a rating of fifty-five or below is said to be low GI because it causes only a little rise in blood sugar levels. Foods considered high GI, fifty-six or above, send blood sugar soaring.

The following are examples of foods that have earned a high GI rating:

— snacks: corn chips, tortilla chips, pretzels, rice cakes;
— foods sweetened with a lot of sugar, honey, molasses, corn syrup, glucose, or dextrose;
— vegetables: parsnips, potatoes (including baked russet potatoes, french fries, fresh mashed potatoes, instant mashed potatoes), corn, beets, carrots;
— fruits: watermelon, raisins, pineapple, cantaloupe, bananas;
— pastas: all thick shapes, including ziti, penne, and rigatoni;
— cereals: old-fashioned oats, corn and most corn products, some rice products, millet, some dry cereals;
— breads: whole wheat bread, cornbread, all baked goods made with white flour.

The following are foods that fall into the low-GI category:

— snacks: cheese, nuts, olives;
— low-fat yogurt
— foods sweetened with sucralose, fructose, saccharine, or aspartame;
— protein foods: unsweetened peanut butter, beans, eggs, unsweetened soy milk;
— fruits: cherries, grapes, apples, peaches, pears, plums, strawberries, oranges, dried apricots;
— vegetables: all except those listed as high GI;
— cereals: rice bran, unsweetened high fiber, all bran cereals;
— pastas: angel hair, linguine, and other thin strands, cellophane noodles, whole grain spaghetti;
— grains: barley, parboiled rice, bulgur, kasha
— breads: pumpernickel, sourdough.

Choosing foods from the low end of the glycemic index can maintain healthy blood sugar and decrease body fat.

When deciding whether or not to eat a particular food, you need to consider the GI in the context of its overall nutritional value. Some high GI foods contain extra fiber as well as vitamins and minerals needed for optimum health. For example, whole wheat bread and white bread have similar GIs, but whole wheat bread is the better choice because of its nutrient content.

The following is a seven-day eating plan of balanced meals that are designed to keep blood sugar at a steady level. The calorie content for each day is between one thousand eight hundred and two thousand, and the carbohydrate content is in the 40 percent range. Familiarizing yourself with the menu will give you an idea of how to balance proteins, fats, and carbohydrates; and you will get used to portion sizes.

Day 1

Breakfast	1 bagel (whole wheat or pumpernickel)
	1 tbsp. cream cheese
	3/4 cup mandarin oranges, drained and mixed with nonfat yogurt
Lunch	2 slices rye bread
	1-oz. package tortilla chips
	2 oz. sliced turkey
	Sliced tomato and lettuce on sandwich
	1 1/4 cups watermelon
	8 oz. skim or 1% milk
	1 tbsp. mustard for sandwich
Snack	8 crackers
Dinner	1 small dinner roll of tortilla
	1/2 cup corn
	4 oz. flank steak, broiled or grilled
	1/2 cup green beans
	1 cup cantaloupe/honeydew melon
	1 tsp. margarine for corn
Eve Snack	1 1/2 cups puffed wheat or rice cereal
	1/2 banana
	8 oz. skim or 1% milk

Day 2

Breakfast
1/2 cup bran flakes cereal
1 slice whole wheat toast
1/2 banana
8 oz. skim or 1% milk
1 tsp. margarine

Lunch
2 slices whole wheat bread
1/2 cup noodles in broth
2 oz. sliced lean ham
carrot sticks
1 apple
8 oz. skim or 1% milk
2 tbsp. reduced-calorie mayonnaise

Snack
3/4 oz. pretzels

Dinner
1 small dinner roll
1/3 cup brown rice
4 oz. baked chicken
1 cup cooked broccoli
1 cup raspberries
1 tsp. margarine
1 tbsp. regular salad dressing with small green salad

Eve Snack
3 cups hot air popcorn
1 small peach
8 oz. sugar-free hot cocoa

Day 3

Breakfast
1 cup pink grapefruit
1 1/4 cups cornflakes
1/2 cup 1% milk
1 slice whole wheat toast
1 oz. cream cheese
1 cup tea

Lunch	3 oz. tuna salad
	2 slices rye bread
	1 red tomato
	1 leaf iceberg lettuce
	1/2 cup canned chickpeas
	1 tbsp. blue cheese dressing
	1 cup 1% milk
	1 pear
	1 cup club soda
Dinner	1/2 breast roast chicken
	1 drumstick
	1 baked potato with skin
	1/2 cup cooked broccoli
	3/4 cup tossed salad
	1 tbsp. Thousand Island dressing
	1 dinner roll
	1 banana
	1 cup tea
Eve Snack	1 apple
	2 melba toast

Day 4

Breakfast	2 fried eggs
	1 slice whole grain bread
	1 tsp. butter
	1/2 cup fat-free milk
	1/2 cup apple juice
Snack	1 nectarine
Lunch	5 oz. grilled chicken tenders
	1 cup salad made with red-leaf lettuce
	1/4 cup shredded carrots
	1/2 cup sliced cucumber
	2 tbsp. Italian dressing
Snack	1 oz. walnuts

Dinner 5	5 oz. London broil
	1 cup green beans
	1/2 cup couscous

| Snack 2 | biscotti cookies |

Day 5

Breakfast	2 scrambled eggs
	1 slice rye toast
	2 tsp. butter
	1/2 cup orange juice
	1/2 cup fat-free milk

| Snack | 1 kiwi fruit |

Lunch	1/2 cup salad made with cooked lentils
	4 oz. turkey breast, cooked and cubed
	1/2 cup sliced carrots
	1/2 cup chopped peppers
	1/4 cup cooked peas
	1 tbsp. olive oil
	1/2 oz. cheddar cheese

| Snack | 1 oz. Brazil nuts |

| Dinner | 5 oz. stir-fried chicken and broccoli |

| Snack | 1 pecan muffin |
| | 2 tsp. butter |

Day 6

Breakfast	1/2 cup cottage cheese
	3/4 cup blueberries
	Pinch cinnamon
	2 slices bacon

| Snack | 15 small grapes |

Lunch	5 oz. lean hamburger
	1/2 whole wheat hamburger bun
	1 leaf lettuce
	1 slice tomato
	1 tsp mustard
	3 tsp. mayonnaise
	10 small french fries
Snack	1 oz. hazelnuts
	1 1/2 oz. reduced-fat cheddar
Dinner	5 oz. cooked turkey breast
	1/2 cup cooked baby carrots
	1/4 cup cooked peas
	2 tsp. olive oil
	1 cup chicken broth soup
Snack	1 peanut butter cookie
	1/2 cup fat-free milk

Day 7

Breakfast	1/2 cup bran cereal flakes
	1/2 cup fat-free milk
	1/2 banana
	1/2 cup cottage cheese
Snack	10 large cherries
	1 protein bar
Lunch	1 serving sausage, egg, and vegetable omelet
	1/2 cup steamed spinach
	1 slice whole wheat bread
Snack	1 oz. almonds
	2 oz. reduced-fat Swiss cheese
Dinner	5 oz. grilled salmon
	1/2 cup steamed asparagus
	1/2 cup cooked brown rice
	1 tsp. butter
Snack	1 oz. pretzels

Oral Hypoglycemics

If you are diagnosed with type II diabetes and medication is necessary to stabilize blood sugars, metformin is one of the best drugs to choose. Metformin (brand name Glucophage) is a new drug that is having a major impact on the treatment of type II diabetes. Since its introduction in the latter part of 1994, it has become a widely prescribed oral hypoglycemics agent. This drug belongs to the class of chemicals called biguanides. Rather than stimulating the production of insulin in the diabetic who may already have high insulin levels, as well as insulin receptors on the cells that do not function normally, this medication sensitizes the body's cells to insulin's effects. In other words, metformin helps the body utilize its own insulin to process the blood sugar more efficiently. Metformin also inhibits gluconeogenesis (the production of glucose from protein and fat) and reduces the release of glucose from the liver. It facilitates the transportation of sugar across the cell membrane and into the cell where it can be used for energy. Because it accomplishes this without stimulating insulin secretion, it lowers blood sugar without the risk of causing hypoglycemia.

Metformin may have some mild side effects. Between 10 percent and 30 percent of those taking the medication experience minimal GI symptoms, which are nausea, vomiting, diarrhea, and anorexia. These symptoms usually subside overtime.

Studies have shown that metformin has a favorable effect on blood lipids and body weight, which is generally stabilized or decreased.

Metformin should not be taken by people who have significant liver disease, kidney disease, or heart failure. It is not recommended for use in alcoholics.

What Is Osteoporosis?

Osteoporosis

Osteoporosis is a debilitating disease that can be prevented and treated. It affects 25 million Americans. Women are four times more likely than men to develop the disease, but men also suffer from osteoporosis.

Sometimes called the "silent disease," osteoporosis often goes undetected until the patient sustains a fracture and seeks medical attention. Osteoporosis is a disease in which bones become fragile and are more likely to break. If not prevented or if left untreated, osteoporosis can progress painlessly until a bone breaks. Any bone can be affected, but the bones of most concern are those of the hip and spine. A hip fracture almost always requires hospitalization and major surgery. It can impair a person's ability to walk unassisted and may cause prolonged or permanent disability or even death. Spinal or vertebral fractures also have serious consequences, including loss of height, severe back pain, and deformity. Each year, osteoporosis is responsible for over seventy thousand hip fractures, fifty thousand wrist fractures, and one hundred twenty thousand spinal fractures.

Who Is at Risk for Getting Osteoporosis?

Everyone is at risk for getting osteoporosis due to the natural decline in bone density that occurs with old age.

Bone is a living tissue that is in a constant state of change. Old, worn-out bone is broken down by cells called osteoclasts and replaced by bone-building cells called osteoblasts. This process is known as remodeling. Usually the breaking down of bone and the subsequent building of new bone are timed so that they occur in close sequence and remain balanced. After the age of thirty, bone loss slightly exceeds bone formation, and overtime, an expected 8-10 percent loss in bone mass will occur. That is why, to prevent osteoporosis, building up as much healthy bone mass as you can, by the time you are thirty, will allow you to lose that 8-10 percent of bone tissue without putting you at risk for bone fractures.

Increased Risk for Women

After menopause, a woman will lose bone six times faster than men for a period of seven to ten years due to a decrease in estrogen. As a woman enters menopause, ovarian function declines. The ovaries are responsible for the production of two hormones—estrogen and progesterone. Estrogen's function is to maintain the normal rate of bone remodeling. When the estrogen levels fall in menopause, bone resorption becomes greater than bone formation, resulting in a net loss of bone. Not all women respond to bone loss during menopause in the same way. The ovaries are not the only source of estrogen. Fat tissue produces androstenediane, which is converted into estrogen. Women who weigh more and have a higher fat content tend to lose less bone in menopause.

What Is Bone Made Of?

Your body is made up of two different types of bones—trabecular bone and cortical bone. Trabecular bone is soft and porous. It is sometimes referred to as spongy bone. It is found in the inner part of most bones and makes up most of your vertebrae, ribs, and sternum.

Cortical bone is the hard outer surface of most bones. Eighty percent of bones are made from cortical bone tissue.

Bone is in a constant state of reformation. Old bone is reabsorbed into the bloodstream, and new bone takes its place. After the cells called osteoclasts break bone down, a cavity is formed. Bone-building cells called osteoblasts immediately start to fill the cavity with new bone. A protein called collagen is the first step in bone formation. Collagen weaves into a matrix to fill the cavity, but it is not yet hardened. The bone will harden by a process called calcification. This occurs by the intake of calcium in your diet. Calcium not only is necessary for strong bones but is needed in every system and process in the body. Muscle contractions, blood clotting, brain function, heart rhythm, and the kidneys all need calcium to work properly. Ninety-five percent of your body's calcium is stored in your bones. Five percent is kept circulating in your blood to assist other body functions. If the calcium level in your blood falls below a certain point, a hormone is released by the parathyroid that will increase the rate of bone resorption (breakdown) so that the calcium level in your blood is maintained at an adequate level. This will lead to increased risk of osteoporosis.

It takes approximately four months for a cycle of remodeling to be completed, and vitamin D is a major factor in bone health. Vitamin D is needed in order for your body to absorb the calcium in your diet. Vitamin D comes into the body through the food we eat and exposure to sunlight. Vitamin D is responsible for the demolition capacity of osteoclasts, the stimulation of bone-building osteoblasts, and the ability of the intestines to absorb the calcium they need to harden the skeleton.

How Is Osteoporosis Diagnosed?

Osteoporosis was called the silent disease because, up until about fifteen years ago, the only way to diagnose the disease was after a fracture had occurred. But today, there are several noninvasive diagnostic tests that can measure a person's bone mass.

The Bone Mineral Density Test. The bone mineral density test is the most current method to measure bone mass. It is based on numbers and allows us to define a fracture threshold for bone mineral density at which point most patients will have a very high risk for developing an osteoporotic fracture. When the bone is measured, several factors will be taken into consideration, including the bone that is measured, the site of interest, and the patient's age and sex.

A value of 2.5 is the cutoff value for osteoporosis. A score of 1 means that a patient's bone mass is 10 percent less than the normal value. A score of 2 means that bone mass is 20 percent less than the normal value. The bone mineral test has allowed for four general categories of bone mass to be established.

The four categories are as follows:

1.   *Normal*—a value for bone mineral density of one or less.
2.   *Low Bone Mass*—a value of bone mineral density of more than 1 but not greater than 2.5. This is also known as osteopenia.
3.   *Osteoporosis*—a value of bone mineral density of more than 2.5.
4.   *Severe Osteoporosis*—a value of bone mineral density more than 2.5 and the presence of one or more osteoporotic fractures.

How Is Bone Mineral Density Level Obtained?

Single Photon Absorptiometry. Single photon absorptiometry (SPA) was the first method to measure bone mass. A densitometer measures the mineral contents of the bones in the forearm by calculating how many gamma rays are absorbed. The greater the absorption, the greater the bone mineral content and the greater the bone mass. The instrument is connected to a computer that reads the results and prints them out onto a graph. SPA measures both types of bone, cortical and trabecular. It is a simple, noninvasive measure of bone mass that has good precision and accuracy.

Dual-Energy X-Ray Absorptiometry. Unlike the SPA, which can only measure bones that are close to the skin's surface, the dual-energy X-ray absorptiometry (DXA) is used for bone sites such as the spine and hip, which are surrounded by muscle, fat, and abdominal organs. The DXA allows us to measure the mass of both superficial and deeper bones.

Ultrasound Measurement of Bone Mass. In ultrasound measurement of bone mass, a quantitative ultrasound device (QUS) measures the speed of a sound wave traveling through the bone. If the bone is thick, the sound wave will travel slowly. If the outside cortical bone is thin and the interior trabecular bone is sparse, the sound will travel quickly. Studies show that the ultrasound measurement gives us different information about bone mass, but is equal to the DXA in predicting future fractures.

Exercises That Prevent Osteoporosis

Peak Bone Mass. Achieving peak bone mass is critical for preventing osteoporosis. The growth begins when you're in the womb and continues through childhood, adolescence, and young adulthood. At about the age of thirty, you have reached your peak bone mass. It is essential for you to achieve the greatest possible density in your bones by the age of thirty.

Diet and exercise are your best resources when reaching peak bone mass. This is called primary prevention. The good news is that there is overwhelming proof that even after you have reached your peak bone mass, diet and exercise can inhibit or reverse bone loss. If you already have osteoporosis, taking steps to increase bone mass and prevent fractures is called secondary prevention.

When we exercise, we put increased stress on the bones. The bones remodel, strengthen, and increase in mass in response to the increased workload. The best exercises to put stress on the skeleton and induce bone formation are weight-bearing exercises. Weight-bearing aerobic exercises include jogging, running, brisk walking, weightlifting, and sports like basketball, baseball, and tennis. It is recommended to do some form of weight-bearing aerobic exercise three to five times a week for thirty minutes. When you start an exercise program, it is important to start slowly and move gradually from one level of difficulty to the next. There are three phases to any weight-bearing exercise session.

1. Warm-up. Start by walking in place for three to five minutes. This brings blood to your muscles and decreases the chance of injury.
2. Perform the exercise you choose. Start at a low level of difficulty and gradually increase the intensity when you feel able. Part 2 should be twenty to thirty minutes in duration.
3. Cool down. Duration is five minutes. This consists of walking slowly. After you have increased your heart rate during exercise, it is important to gradually decrease the rate of your pulse to prevent blood pooling in the legs. Walking around slowly for five minutes will achieve this.

The second form of exercise you will do to increase the strength of your muscles and put increased stress on your bones is weight training. You will do several individual exercises with the use of hand weights. The recommended starting weight for women is 1.5-3 pounds and progresses to five-pound hand weights, progressing to ten and fifteen pounds.

When you begin a weight training workout, it is important to begin with a warm-up of three to five minutes. This will get your heart pumping blood to your muscles and reduces the chance that you will injure yourself during the exercise program.

Weight training is done with repetitions and sets. A repetition is a repeating of an exercise for a designated number of times in a row, without a rest. A set refers to a group of repetitions. If more than one set of an exercise is supposed to be performed, then you should take a short rest of one to two minutes between each set.

For example, if an exercise calls for three sets of eight-to-twelve repetitions, that means, you repeat the exercise eight to twelve times in a row. Then you rest for a minute or two. Then do the second set of eight-to-twelve repetitions. Rest a minute or two, and finally, do the exercise again (third set) for another eight-to-twelve repetitions.

Start with a weight training program of a five-to-ten-minute workout three times a week, and then slowly work up to a minimum of twenty minutes two to three times a week.

The following are the exercises you will do in a weight training program.

Exercise 1—Bench Press

Lie on your back with your feet flat on the floor or on a bench. Hold the hand weights against your upper chest in each hand. Your hands should be shoulder-width apart, with the palms facing toward your feet and your back flat on the bench. Push the weights straight up until your arms are fully extended. Then bring down the weights slowly to the starting position with the weights against your upper chest. This exercise builds up the muscles in your chest and arms.

Exercise 2—Frontal-Lateral Raises

Stand with your feet shoulder-width apart, stomach tight, back straight, and knees slightly bent. Start with your hands in front of your thighs and with your arms slightly bent. Lift the weights directly in front of you to shoulder height, palms down. Slowly return the weights to starting position. This exercise builds up the shoulder muscles.

Exercise 3—Lateral-Side Raises

Stand with your feet shoulder-width apart, abs tight, back straight, and knees slightly bent. Hold weights at your side. Raise the weights out to your sides. Arms should be straight and palms down. Return to the starting position. Do three sets of eight-to-twelve repetitions, resting one to two minutes in between sets. This exercise works the shoulders.

Exercise 4—Overhead Presses

Sit in a chair with your back straight and your abs tight. Start with the weights in your hands at shoulder level, palms forward. Exhale as you press the weights directly over your head until your arms are straight. Slowly lower the weights to the starting position and repeat. Do three sets of eight-to-twelve repetitions, resting one minute in between sets. This exercise works the shoulders.

Exercise 5—Standing Dumbbell Curls

Stand upright with your knees slightly bent to give you support. Hold a dumbbell (weight) in each hand with an underhand grip and your forearms turned toward the front. Raise both dumbbells to the tops of your shoulders, always holding your body steady through the movement. Your elbows should remain stationary as a kind of pivot point just above your hips. Then slowly lower the weights to the starting position. This exercise strengthens the bicep muscles. Do three sets of eight-to-twelve repetitions, resting one to two minutes in between sets.

Exercise 6—Upright Rows

Stand with your feet wider than your shoulders. Your abs should be tight, and your knees slightly bent. Hold the weights with your palms facing in. Raise the weights so your arms form the letter V. Inhale as you lift, squeezing your shoulder blades together, then return your arms to the starting position and repeat. Do three sets of eight-to-twelve repetitions each. Rest thirty seconds in between sets. This exercise works the upper back.

Exercise 7—Lunges

Stand with your feet together and a dumbbell in each hand at your sides. Your arms should be fully extended downward with your palms pointing toward your body. Step forward, bending your stepping leg in a lunge movement, with the knee bent as though you were lowering yourself to the floor. The back leg should be kept straight at the knee. Then, push your body back up to the starting position by using only the muscles of the bent leg. Keep your back straight throughout the exercise. Then repeat the movement using the opposite leg. When you have done a lunge on each leg, count that as one repetition. Do three sets of eight-to-twelve repetitions, resting one minute in between sets. This exercise works the thighs, buttocks, and hamstrings.

Exercise 8—Leg Lift

Lie on your left side, with your left leg extended straight down, in-line with your body. Position your right leg directly out in front at a ninety-degree angle to your body. Support your body by placing your hands and left elbow firmly on the floor in front of your chest and head. Raise your right leg toward the ceiling without bending your knee. Keep your right foot flexed toward the ceiling during the movement. When you've completed the required number of sets and repetitions with the right leg, turn over onto your right side and repeat the exercise using your left leg. Do three sets of eight-to-twelve repetitions, resting one minute in between sets. This exercise works the outer thigh.

Exercise 9—Rear Leg Lift

Kneel with your elbows and knees on the floor. Keeping the left leg bent, extend your right leg straight back and raise it toward the ceiling as far as you can. Then return your right leg to the starting position. When you have finished the required number of sets and repetitions for the right leg, go through these same movements with the left leg. This exercise strengthens the muscles of the back of the leg and the lower back. Do three sets of eight-to-twelve repetitions, waiting one minute in between sets.

Exercise 10—Scissor-Leg Lift

Lie on your left side, with your left leg straight down in-line with your body. Bend your right knee and place your right foot behind the knee of your left leg. Supporting yourself with your hands and elbows, raise your right leg straight upward and then return your right leg to the starting position. Repeat this movement for three sets of eight-to-twelve repetitions, waiting one minute in between sets. Change to the right side and repeat. This exercise works the muscles in your legs, hips, abdomen, and lower back.

Calcium from Food Sources

It is recommended that a person get an average calcium intake of between 1,200 mg and 1,500 mg daily. This dosage is optimum for bone health. In addition to calcium, an adequate amount of vitamin D must be included in the diet in order for calcium to be absorbed properly in the small intestines.

If the suggested amount of calcium cannot be obtained daily through food sources, a supplement is strongly encouraged.

The following chart is a list of foods high in calcium content.

Food	Amount	Calcium (mg)
Green Leafy Vegetables		
1. Collard greens	1 cup	300 mg
2. Broccoli	1 cup	450 mg
3. Kale	1 cup	179 mg
4. Spinach	1 cup	278 mg
5. Turnip greens	1 cup	229 mg
6. Beet greens	1 cup	165 mg
7. Bok choy	1 cup	200 mg
8. Mustard greens	1 cup	150 mg
9. Rhubarb	1 cup	348 mg
10. Parsley (raw)	1 cup	122 mg
Fish		
1. Sardines	3 1/2-oz. can	300 mg
2. Salmon (canned)	1 cup	431 mg
3. Oysters (raw)	1 cup	226 mg
Beans and Legumes		
1. Tofu	4 oz.	80-150 mg
2. Chickpeas	1 cup (cooked)	150 mg
3. Black beans	1 cup (cooked)	135 mg
4. Pinto beans	1 cup (cooked)	128 mg
Dairy		
1. Milk		
Milk	1 cup	300 mg
Whole	1 cup	288 mg
2. Cheese		
(American, Swiss, cheddar)	1 1/2 oz.	300 mg
3. Ice milk	1 cup	204 mg
4. Nonfat yogurt	1 cup	294 mg
5. Cottage cheese (low fat)	1 cup	150 mg

Nuts and Seeds

1.	Sesame seeds	3 tbsp.	300 mg
2.	Almonds	1 cup	300 mg
3.	Sunflower seeds	1 cup	174 mg
4.	Brazil nuts	1 cup	260 mg
5.	Hazel nuts	1 cup	282 mg

Fortified Juice and Water

1.	Orange juice (Minute Maid)	1 cup	210 mg
2.	Perrier water	1 liter	140 mg
3.	Mendocino	1 liter	380 mg
4.	San Pellegrino	1 liter	200 mg

Hormone-Replacement Therapy

Osteoporosis and Menopause

As we discussed earlier, during menopause, a woman loses bone mass at a rate of seven times faster than usual due to the loss of estrogen production from the ovaries. Hormone replacement therapy (HRT) involves the use of estrogen, either alone or in combination with progesterone hormones. Because estrogen used alone involves the risk of uterine and other cancers, progestins have been added to recent formulas. Progestins, taken either together with estrogen or on alternative days, usually remove the risk of developing uterine cancer. It is very important for a woman to know her own risk of cancer based on her family history.

It is clear that the woman who uses estrogen alone for a long time runs an increased risk of developing cancer of the endometrium. The risk in women who have used estrogen alone, compared to women who have never used estrogen, is about two times higher. This effect increases with the number of years of therapy and with higher doses of estrogen.

It has been proven that the women who have taken estrogen have a small increase in the risk for acquiring breast cancer. A recent study found that fifteen years of estrogen use might increase the risk of breast cancer by about one and a half times compared to the risk of a woman who has never taken estrogen.

The Benefits of Hormone Replacement Therapy (HRT)

Women who start hormone replacement therapy and continue it for seven to ten years will gain long-term protection against an osteoporotic fracture. In one study, which included both healthy postmenopausal women and women who have had their ovaries removed, estrogen treatments were given for two to six years after the ovaries ceased to function. As a result, the women experienced an average of 1-3 percent rise per year in bone density in their arms and legs.

Many other studies consistently show that hormone replacement therapy reduces the risk of osteoporotic fractures of the hip and the forearm by about 30-40 percent and the risk of fractures of the spine by over 50 percent. The longer a woman takes estrogen after menopause, the lower her risk of suffering an osteoporotic fracture.

The benefits of HRT are obvious, but due to the controversy of developing certain cancers, it should be used with caution and only for severe cases of bone loss.

Medications Approved for Increasing Bone Mass

Raloxifene (Evista) is approved for prevention and treatment of postmenopausal osteoporosis. The drug reduces bone turnover and thereby increases bone mass density. For maximal benefits, treatment must be accompanied by adequate intake of calcium and vitamin D.

In the MORE (Multiple Outcomes of Raloxifene Evaluation) trial, treatment with raloxifene (60 or 120 mg once a day) for thirty-six months increased bone mass density and reduced the risk of fractures. The increase in bone mass density was 2.31 in the femoral neck of the hip and 3.71 in the spine. Increased bone mass density was associated with a reduced risk of spinal fractures. After thirty-six months, at least one new spinal fracture was seen in 10.1 percent of the women taking placebo, compared with 6.61 percent of those taking 60 mg of raloxifene and 5.41 of those taking 129 mg of raloxifene. This represents a 52 percent decrease in risk with raloxifene.

Alendronate (Fosamax). At this time, alendronate (Fosamax) is the only bisphosphanate approved for postmenopausal osteoporosis. The drug is safe and prevents fractures. Alendronate was approved initially only for treating existing osteoporosis and was later approved for osteoporosis prevention. In both cases, benefits derive from inhibiting bone resorption by osteoclasts. To be effective, alendronate must be accompanied by adequate intake of calcium and vitamin D.

When studied in osteoporotic postmenopausal women (average age of sixty-five), alendronate produced a modest increase in bone mass density in the hip and spine. More importantly, treatment decreased the rate of new fractures. Compared with patients taking placebo, those taking alendronate experienced 51 percent fewer fractures of the hip, 47 percent fewer fractures of the spine, and 48 percent fewer fractures of the wrist. Furthermore, when spinal fractures did occur, loss of height was less than in women who got spinal fractures while taking placebo. The dosage for treatment of osteoporosis is 10 mg daily.

When given to prevent osteoporosis in postmenopausal women (ages forty-four to fifty), alendronate produced a small increase in BMD of the spine and hip. In contrast, women taking placebo lost bone mass density at both sites. The response to alendronate was basically the same as the response to estrogen. The dosage for prevention of osteoporosis is 5 mg a day—half the dosage used to treat osteoporosis.

What Is Heart Disease?

Heart Disease

Heart disease is the leading cause of death in men and women of all ethnic and racial groups in the United States. Almost one in every four Americans has one or more types of heart disease. Heart disease is any disease of the heart and the circulatory system.

High Blood Pressure

There are several different types of heart disease. The most common and preventable types are hypertension (high blood pressure) and coronary artery disease.

High blood pressure (hypertension) is our most common chronic illness. The American Heart Association estimates that approximately 35-40 million people suffer from the disease. High blood pressure is the leading cause of strokes and a major risk factor for heart attacks. High blood pressure is called the silent killer. You can have it and not even know it. High blood pressure seldom causes symptoms that warn you of a problem. High blood pressure is a serious condition; and if left undetected, it can damage your circulatory system, including the blood vessels of your heart, brain, eyes, and kidneys. The higher the pressure or the longer it goes undetected, the worse the prognosis.

Each time your heart beats, two or three ounces of freshly oxygenated blood are forced out of the heart and through the circulatory system that consists of sixty thousand miles of blood vessels. The circulatory system branches off from large vessels to smaller ones. The smallest blood vessels, known as the capillaries, are the microscopic vessels that supply blood full of oxygen and other nutrients to each cell in the body.

A certain level of force is needed to keep blood moving through the blood vessels. The amount of force that is exerted on the artery walls as blood flows through them is what we call blood pressure. The more your heart pumps and the smaller the arteries, the higher your blood pressure (i.e., the harder your heart must work to pump the same amount of blood).

The standard way to measure blood pressure is in millimeters of mercury (mmHg). This unit of measurement refers to how high the pressure inside your arteries is able to raise a column of mercury. Each blood pressure measurement has two numbers and is written like a fraction. The top number is your systolic blood pressure, or the highest pressure within your arteries that occurs during systole, when your heart is contracting. The bottom number is your diastolic blood pressure, or the lowest pressure within your arteries that occurs during diastole, when your heart is relaxing and filling with blood.

Diagnosing High Blood Pressure

Blood pressure is measured with a device called a sphygmomanometer, which consists of an inflatable rubber cuff, an air pump, and a column of mercury or a dial or digital readout reflecting pressure in an air column. The cuff is wrapped around the upper arm, and the inflatable cuff is tightened until blood flow through the large artery in the arm is momentarily stopped. As air is pumped into the cuff, it pushes up a column of mercury.

The person measuring the blood pressure places a stethoscope over the artery just below the cuff and listens for a cessation of the sound of blood flowing through the artery. He or she then begins to release air from the cuff, allowing blood to flow through the artery again. As air is released, the column of mercury or air begins to fall, and the person listens for the first thumping sound that signals a return of blood flow into the vessel over which the stethoscope has been placed. The height of the column of mercury or air pressure on the dial at this sound indicates the systolic (or higher) pressure. More air is released from the cuff, and the pressure continues to fall. The height of the mercury or the level of air pressure when the thumping sound of blood stops, indicating the pause between heartbeats, is the diastolic pressure.

Blood pressure varies during the course of an average day. The average blood pressure in an adult is 120/80 mmHg.

Either your diastolic pressure or your systolic pressure—or both—may be elevated. Elevated diastolic pressure promotes damage to your kidneys and to blood vessels throughout your body. High systolic blood pressure is associated with a higher risk of coronary artery disease or stroke.

High blood pressure should not be based on a single reading. Several readings, done at different times, are needed to confirm an accurate diagnosis of high blood pressure. Hypertension is typically defined as readings higher than 140/90 mmHg (measured in millimeters of mercury). This cutoff was chosen to define high blood pressure because the risk of cardiovascular complication becomes very significant at this point.

There are several classifications of blood pressure. The following chart outlines the ranges for normal and hypertensive readings.

Diastolic Readings

Range in mmHg

Diastolic	*Diagnosis*	*Recommendation*
Below 85	Normal blood pressure	Recheck within 2 years.
85-89	High normal blood pressure	Recheck within 1 year.
90-144	Mild hypertension	Confirm within 2 months.
105-114	Moderate hypertension	Therapy needs to be taken.
Above 115	Severe hypertension	Begin therapy with medication.

Systolic Hypertension

Below 140	Normal blood pressure	Recheck within 2 years.
140-159	Borderline systolic hypertension	Confirm within 2 months.
160-199	Systolic hypertension	Confirm within 2 months. Therapy should be started if pressure remains elevated.
Above 200	Systolic hypertension	Begin therapy with medication.

What Causes High Blood Pressure?

Think of your blood vessels like a tube. If the tube is clear, with no particles stuck along the walls of it, blood flow remains at a smooth, constant pressure. But if for some reason the tube has become narrow, the flow of blood meets resistance, and the pressure goes up.

Over 90 percent of high blood pressure cases have no identifiable cause. The elevated blood pressure in this case is referred to as primary or essential hypertension. It is believed that this type of high blood pressure may be due to hormonal factors relating to the handling of salt by the kidneys and/or to the elaboration of certain substances that cause constriction of blood vessels. These are probably genetically determined, but environmental factors such as a high-salt, low-potassium diet and chronic stress may play some roles.

For the other 10 percent of patients, high blood pressure could be the result of another disorder or a side effect of medication. This type of hypertension is referred to as secondary hypertension. These cases are relatively uncommon.

Who Is at Risk for Getting High Blood Pressure?

High blood pressure develops in all social and economic groups and affects both men and women. It generally begins in adulthood between the ages of thirty-five and fifty, although it also occurs to a lesser extent among children and younger adults.

Some people are more susceptible to acquiring hypertension than others. These include:

African Americans. African Americans are twice likely to develop high blood pressure than whites, and their disease is also more severe.

People with Diabetes. High blood pressure is much more common in individuals with diabetes than it is in the general population. It is also particularly dangerous for them because it carries a high risk of cardiovascular complications. It is thought by researchers that the elevated sugar levels damage the walls of the blood vessels, increasing resistance of blood pressure and thus causing hypertension.

People Who Are Overweight. If you are overweight, your risk for developing high blood pressure is two to six times what it would be if you maintained a healthy weight. As you put on weight, you gain mostly fatty tissue. Just like other parts of your body, this tissue relies on oxygen and nutrients in your blood to survive. As the demand for oxygen and nutrients increases, the amount of blood circulating through your body also increases. More blood traveling through your arteries means added pressure on your artery walls. Weight gain also typically increases the level of insulin in your blood—an increase associated with retention of sodium and water, which increases blood volume.

People with a Family History of the Disease. Babies born to parents who have hypertension tend to have higher-than-average blood pressures throughout infancy and childhood and are more likely to develop hypertension at an early age. This strongly suggests that there is a genetic basis for at least some cases of high blood pressure. It does not mean, however, that if both parents have hypertension, the child or the parents will always develop high blood pressure.

Population studies suggest a number of other factors that may increase the risk of having high blood pressure. These include consuming large amounts of salt (sodium) and alcohol (more than three to four ounces of alcohol daily), smoking cigarettes, and following a diet low in potassium. It is not exactly understood how these factors raise blood pressure, but some people appear to be more susceptible to them than others. For example, a high-salt diet may raise blood pressure only in people who have a genetic tendency to conserve sodium. Similarly, many people who consume excessive amounts of alcohol have normal blood pressures.

Long-Term Complications of High Blood Pressure

Hypertension is called the silent killer because it does not produce definite symptoms until it reaches an advanced stage. Untreated high blood pressure is the major cause of strokes; it is also one of the major risk factors for a heart attack. Even if a person is feeling well with hypertension, if left untreated, high blood pressure is causing damage to vital organs throughout the body. The good news is that the long-term complications of high blood pressure can be prevented by lowering the blood pressure into the normal range and keeping it there.

Blood Vessels

High blood pressure speeds up the process of hardening of the arteries in both large blood vessels and the smaller ones. The increased pressure on the inner walls of the blood vessels makes them more vulnerable to a buildup of fatty deposits, a condition called atherosclerosis. This blood vessel damage may not produce symptoms until it reaches an advanced stage. If the blood vessels to the heart begin to narrow and the heart muscle is unable to get enough blood, angina (chest pains) will occur. Narrowed arteries in the lower legs can cause pain when walking. This condition is called intermittent claudication.

Blood clots are more likely to form in arteries that have been narrowed by deposits of fatty material. A clot in a blood vessel going to the heart can cause a heart attack. A clot obstructing blood supply to the brain can result in a stroke.

High blood pressure also damages the small arteries. The muscles that form the lining of these vessels and obstructing blood flow through them. If this happens, parts of the body that are supplied with blood by these small vessels can become damaged—such as the kidneys and the eyes.

The Kidneys

Each day, more than four hundred gallons of blood flow through the kidneys. The main function of the kidneys is to filter waste products and excrete them out in the urine and to return nutrients and other useful substances back into the bloodstream. Continuous high blood pressure forces the kidneys to work even harder. This increased pressure will eventually damage some of the tiny blood vessels within the kidney and reduce the amount of blood available to the filtering nephrons. After a period of time, their ability to filter the blood efficiently is reduced. As a result, uremia may develop. Uremia is an accumulation of waste products in the blood that are normally eliminated in the urine but, due to the damaged filtering system of the kidneys, are unable to be excreted as waste. Uremia is a serious condition eventually leading to kidney failure, a condition requiring periodic dialysis to cleanse the blood.

The Heart

As you know, the heart needs a constant supply of fresh, oxygenated blood to sustain life. High blood pressure forces the heart to work harder to supply an adequate amount of blood flow to the tissues, resulting in an enlarged heart. The heart is a muscle, and any increased strain on a muscle will make it become larger. As time goes on, the enlarged heart becomes stiff and weak and unable to pump efficiently. This can lead to heart failure, a condition in which the heart is unable to pump enough blood to meet the body's needs. Heart failure today can generally be controlled with medications, allowing most patients to live normal lives for many years. The best news is recent studies show that with effective treatment of high blood pressure, much of the heart enlargement can actually be reversed.

The Eyes

The eyes contain tiny blood vessels that are susceptible to damage from high blood pressure. The retina, which is located in the back of the eye, may sustain hemorrhages and/or fat deposits due to compromised blood supply. This condition is referred to as retinopathy. If this situation occurs, diminished vision and blindness can occur. However, due to the advances in controlling high blood pressure, these situations are increasingly uncommon.

The Brain

The brain needs a constant supply of oxygen and nutrients supplied by the blood. If the vessels that supply blood to the brain become clogged with fatty deposits, blood flow to the brain may become compromised. If this situation occurs, the risk of a stroke is greatly increased. A stroke is the interruption of blood flow to the brain; that is a life-threatening situation. It can result in permanent brain damage or even death.

Medicines That Treat
High Blood Pressure

Medicines are necessary whenever positive lifestyle changes haven't succeeded enough to bring blood pressure to a normal level.

There are three general classes of medications used in controlling high blood pressure:

Diuretics. Diuretics lower blood pressure by lowering blood volume through increasing the amount of sodium and water excreted through the kidneys.

Alpha Blockers and Beta Blockers. These medications inhibit various portions of the nervous system, particularly receptors called alpha and beta receptors. Inhibiting them helps lower blood pressure by slowing the heart rate and decreasing the force with which the heart pumps or by helping arteries to relax or dilate, thus lowering the pressure required to pump blood through the arteries.

Vasodilators. Vasodilators act directly on the walls of the arteries and cause them to relax, reducing the amount of pressure needed to pump blood through the arteries. There are two major types of vasodilators:

— *ACE Inhibitors*: These drugs help reduce blood pressure by decreasing substances in the blood that cause vessels to constrict. The acronym "ACE" stands for angiotensin-converting enzyme. Both short-acting (taken several times a day) and long-acting (taken once a day) ACE inhibitors are available for treatment of high blood pressure.

— *Calcium Antagonists*: Also called calcium channel blockers, calcium antagonists inhibit the inward flow of calcium into cardiac and blood vessel tissues, thereby reducing the tension of the heart and the constriction of blood vessels.

Preventing High Blood Pressure

Although doctors don't know the exact mechanisms that cause primary hypertension, a number of conditions are strongly associated with increases in high blood pressure. Taking away any one of these risk factors usually leads to lower blood pressure, and for many, controlling these conditions actually returns their blood pressure to normal levels.

Physical Inactivity

People who are physically inactive increase their likelihood of developing high blood pressure. In one large study of more than sixteen thousand individuals, inactive people were 35 percent more likely to develop hypertension than were active people, regardless of whether they had a family history of high blood pressure.

Maintaining a Moderate Alcohol Intake

There is some evidence that a moderate intake of alcohol may actually help lower the risk of cardiovascular disease. There is also evidence that an intake of more than three ounces of alcohol a day may increase the risk of developing high blood pressure or cardiovascular disease. The Joint National Committee on Detection, Evaluation, and Treatment of High Blood Pressure recommends that people should drink "no more than one ounce of ethanol a day." This amount is contained in two ounces of 100-proof whiskey, about eight ounces of wine or about twenty-four ounces of beer.

Alcohol in moderation is acceptable in most people. In a number of cases, blood pressure has become easy to control once patients have reduced their excessive intakes of alcohol.

Cigarette Smoking

Cigarette smoking and the use of other tobacco products increase blood pressure both in the short-term while you are smoking and in the long-term because components in the smoke, such as nicotine, cause your arteries to constrict. As we mentioned before, when an artery becomes narrow, resistance increases and blood pressure rises.

Obesity

Hypertension is clearly associated with obesity (weighing more than 20 percent above your desirable body weight). Obesity contributes to an estimated 40 percent or more of all high blood pressure cases in the United States. Losing excess weight will normalize blood pressure. A commonsense diet that reduces the intake of total calories and fats (especially saturated fats) and emphasizes complex carbohydrates and protein as the major diet components may help reduce weight and control many of the risk factors that predispose people to early cardiovascular disease.

Reducing Sodium Intake

A major theory about what causes essential hypertension is the problem that your kidneys appear to have with handling excess salt. Population studies show that societies in which people consume large amounts of salt (such as the United States) have a correspondingly high incidence of high blood pressure. Similarly, in cultures where salt intake is low, the incidence of high blood pressure is extremely low. Other studies show that for most people with hypertension, restricting salt intake helps lower high blood pressure.

Coronary Artery Disease

Coronary artery disease, also known as atherosclerosis, is another type of heart disease that is highly preventable. It is the slow, progressive narrowing of the three main arteries (and their branches) that supply blood to the heart. This narrowing of the arteries gradually starves the heart muscle of the high level of oxygenated blood that it needs to function properly. A lack of adequate blood supply to the heart produces symptoms that range from angina to heart attack or sudden death.

Fatty deposits called plaque, or lesions, build up on the interior walls, narrowing the arteries. Other substances such as cholesterol, fats, cellular wastes, platelets, and calcium also contribute to the closure of the artery. These deposits usually start with fatty streaks and grow to large bumps that distort the artery and block its interior where the blood must flow.

What Causes Coronary Artery Disease?

There are three major factors that play a role in the disease process of atherosclerosis:

Elevated cholesterol and lipids. When blood levels of cholesterol, particularly LDL (low-density lipoprotein) cholesterol, are too high, excess LDL cholesterol is deposited on the endothelial lining of arteries. This trapped LDL can damage the cells by a process called oxidation. The oxidation attracts certain protective cells already in artery walls and circulating in the blood that engulf the oxidized excess lipids. Soon other protective mechanisms such as platelets, T cells, and growth factors for smooth muscle cells are working hard to restore the damage from excess lipid. Unfortunately, this process, which is intended to restore the artery wall to normal, overdoes it. As the process seals off the excess lipids, it creates cholesterol-rich pockets covered with scar tissue. These lesions narrow arteries and typically deform artery walls as they grow larger.

Chronic injury to the endothelium. Damage to the endothelium, or lining of the artery walls, is largely the result of the action of such risk factors as high blood pressure, smoking, and elevated levels of cholesterol and other lipids in the blood. This damage gives cholesterol and other cells that eventually form plaques a way to attach to the endothelium lining or enter the artery walls. It also appears to cause inflammation and activate the cellular-repair crew of the immune system, which speeds to injury sites.

Inflammation. From its earliest stages, atherosclerosis appears to trigger inflammation, the body's first line of defense against injury and infection. Evidence suggests that inflammation serves as a mediator in the disease progression by recruiting various immune system repair-and-fighter cells. Researchers have long suspected that inflammation contributes to atherosclerosis. In addition to attracting substances that narrow the artery walls, inflammation may weaken the surface of the atherosclerotic plaques and thereby increase the risk of plaque rupture.

Symptoms of Coronary Artery Disease (CAD)

The primary symptom of coronary artery disease is chest pain or angina. A person suffering from angina may clutch a fist to the chest while describing a feeling of discomfort or pain, often using such words as "pressure" or "heaviness." This pain is usually located in the center of the chest but may radiate to or occur only in the neck, shoulder, arm, or lower jaw, particularly on the left side.

For most people, these symptoms almost always occur during or after physical activity and/or emotional stress and are more likely to occur following a meal or in cold weather.

Angina may be more likely to occur following a meal because blood rushes to the stomach and the intestinal tract to aid digestion, increasing the work of the heart.

Angina symptoms usually fade and disappear when the person stops the particular activity that brought them on.

Cardiac Catheterization

Cardiac catheterization, also called cath or angiography, often is used to make the final diagnosis of CAD when other tests have suggested that it is present. By taking actual pictures of the arteries when contrast material is injected into them, cardiac catheterization provides direct evidence, whether narrowings are present and provides the physician with a road map that helps guide the patients and physician in determining the next steps in the treatment of CAD whenever it is present.

Diagnosing Angina

A patient's own description of chest pain he or she experiences provides the most important information leading to the diagnosis of angina. In addition, there are several tests that are used to confirm the condition.

Stress Echocardiogram. An echocardiogram taken at rest and then during exercise or drug-simulated exercise can provide evidence of inadequate blood flow to the heart by showing images of the normal or abnormal motions of the heart muscle as it contracts.

Electrocardiogram. ECG or EKG tracings made by an ECG machine during an episode of chest pain can show a number of characteristic changes that can help a physician make the diagnosis of angina.

Preventing Coronary Artery Disease

Many of the same principles for preventing high blood pressure also apply to the prevention of CAD. They are:

1. Maintaining a healthy body weight
2. Increasing physical activity
3. Quitting smoking

But in addition to these risk factors, managing your cholesterol through improved nutrition and, in some cases, medications may be necessary.

Cholesterol

Cholesterol is one of several types of fats (lipids) that play important roles in your body. It is an important component of cell membranes and, therefore, vital to the structure and function of all cells in your body. Cholesterol is also a building block in the formation of certain types of hormones.

However, cholesterol is also the predominant substance in atherosclerotic plaques, which may develop in your arteries and impede the flow of blood. When the cholesterol level in your bloodstream becomes excessively high, the likelihood of your developing atherosclerotic plaques increases.

Cholesterol is measured by a simple blood test. Lipid-level goals are:

Total cholesterol	Less than 200 mg/dl
Total triglycerides	Less than 200 mg/dl
HDL cholesterol	More than 35 mg/dl
LDL cholesterol	Less than 130 mg/dl

If your total cholesterol is over 200 or your HDL is less than 35 and your LDL is greater than 130, you and your doctor will need to discuss a plan in order to get your cholesterol levels in the appropriate range.

Let's Get Moving!

Your Thirty-Day Weight Loss and Fitness Program

Congratulations! You did it!

You took the first step that will change the rest of your life. My thirty-day weight loss and fitness program will empower you to have more energy and enthusiasm for life on an everyday basis. On our journey together, you will cleanse your body of toxins; and the exercise segment will help boost your metabolism to burn fat, lose weight, and give you more energy to live your life and make you feel happier every day. There's a saying—and it is very true—"Look better, feel better, do better!"

And there's more! As you read in the first section of the book, diet and exercise play a major role in the prevention of many debilitating diseases. Not only will you look great and feel incredible, but you will be helping yourself live a long and healthy life. What could be better?

In 1966, the U.S. Surgeon General's Report on physical activity and health was a call to encourage more Americans to become active. The report states that by becoming moderately active, Americans can lower their risk of premature death and the development of chronic illnesses such as heart disease, hypertension, and diabetes. (I would also like to add osteoporosis—brittle bones.) Among its major findings were the following points:

- People who are usually inactive can improve their health and well-being by becoming even *moderately* active on a regular basis.
- Physical activity does not need to be strenuous to achieve health benefits.
- Enhanced fitness and physiological changes occur when the amount (frequency, intensity, and duration) of the activity is increased.

Guidelines from the Surgeon General's Report include the following:

- Acquire thirty minutes of moderate activity on most, if not all, days of the week.
- A moderate amount of physical activity uses approximately 150 calories per day or one thousand calories per week.

It has been medically proven that exercise and nutrition are your best defense against becoming chronically ill.

The plan is thirty days because it takes thirty days for your subconscious mind to engrave a new habit into its system. Most of the reasons why we do not eat right, drink enough water, and exercise are the results of bad habits. Your subconscious mind is programmed to do these bad habits. So it will take a conscious effort to undo them and reprogram your mind with positive lifestyle changes.

I have mapped out your next thirty days with healthy eating suggestions, exercises, and motivational tips. All you need to do is follow the daily "recipe for success," and your subconscious mind will kick in and make these new habits your own.

In today's world, women and men wear many different hats. We are mothers and fathers, employees, wives and husbands. The stress level is high, and that is why it is so important to take time for you. This plan is yours. Give it to yourself, because you can't take care of anyone else unless you take good care of yourself first! Having more energy for life, looking great, reducing stress, and preventing disease are what this plan will do.

Disease is the result of a part of the body not getting the nutrients it needs. One of the best ways to make sure that your body is fully functioning is to aerobically exercise. When you are exercising aerobically, you are increasing your heart rate. The heart muscle is exercised to beat faster so that it can pump blood to every cell in the body and give it the oxygen it needs to perform respiration on a cellular level. At the same time, the lungs are breathing in fresh oxygen and ridding the body of carbon dioxide. The fresh oxygen is carried by the blood throughout the entire body. The result: disease prevention.

There are so many parts to the human body. If a person does not exercise and eats a diet of foods high in saturated fats, the circulatory system (blood vessels) are moving at a sluggish rate and may have blockages in the vessels (fat deposits). If this occurs, areas in your body may not be getting all the nutrients they need to function properly. Each and every cell in your body carries on cellular respiration. Each cell has a life of its own. It needs food and water, and it needs to rid itself of waste. If it does not get the energy it needs and waste builds up, it will start to die or mutate into an abnormal cell, and disease will occur.

Aerobic exercise will prevent this from happening. By exercising the heart thirty minutes a day, five times a week, every cell in your body will receive fresh, oxygenated blood and will release waste from it that will travel through the bloodstream and will be eliminated from the body through your gastrointestinal system, sweat in the skin, or lungs as carbon dioxide. The result is that you are ridding your body of toxins and ensuring that each cell in your body is functioning at its optimum level—and you will feel fantastic!

Let's Get Started!

Every exercise program includes three components: cardiorespiratory fitness, strength training and flexibility.

Cardiorespiratory Fitness

Cardiorespiratory fitness uses the aerobic energy system. Aerobic means air. It is defined as the ability to perform repetitive, moderate-to-high-intensity, large-muscle movements for a prolonged period of time using oxygen. Cardiorespiratory exercise is the most efficient way to reduce weight because it uses fat for fuel. There are also several other benefits to this form of exercise, including:

- stronger heart
- lowered blood pressure
- increased high-density lipoprotein
- stronger bones
- improved sleep
- decreased body fat
- increased ability to perform work with less fatigue
- increased cardiac output
- improved cholesterol ratio
- decreased stress
- decreased depression
- improved immune system
- improved glucose tolerance and insulin sensitivity
- improved quality of life
- decreased resting heart rate
- increase metabolism
- increased endurance, stamina, and energy
- increased ability to metabolize fat

To be effective, aerobic workouts depend on three variables: frequency, intensity, and duration.

Frequency

A frequency of three to five days per week is recommended. If you are trying to lose those extra pounds, four to five days a week are better than three. A beginner should start by doing three days a week, and if that person has not exercised in a long time and is "deconditioned," they can do several small bouts of ten-minute segments.

Intensity

Intensity is a very important component to aerobic exercise. The total amount of work performed is one of the most significant factors in improving cardiorespiratory fitness. Low-to-moderate-intensity training programs with longer durations are recommended for most adults. This decreases the risk of injury and increases adherence (sticking with it).

How to Figure Out the Right Intensity for You

There are two methods that we will use to find your correct intensity of aerobic exercise. The first is the HR method. This method is very simple and is used in most health clubs.

Take the number 220 and subtract your age. That will give you your estimated maximal heart rate. A person needs to work at an intensity of 50-85 percent of their maximal heart rate to achieve the benefits of cardiorespiratory training.

Example 1

1. 220 - age = estimated maximal heart rate
2. Estimated maximal heart rate x percentage (e.g. 70 percent) = target heart rate.

To take your heart rate, palpate the radial artery at your wrist with your forefinger and index finger. Once you find your pulse, count the number of beats for one full minute (or you can count the number of beats for ten seconds and multiply by six). This will give you your heart rate.

Example 2

Let's say you are forty years old and want to work at an intensity of 75 percent of heart rate maximum:

1. 220 - 40 = 180 (estimated heart rate maximum)
2. 180 x 0.75 = 135 BPM (beats per minute)

Immediately after aerobically exercising, take your pulse for one minute, either by counting beats for a full minute or by taking your pulse for ten seconds and multiplying it by six. Your heart rate should be at 135 to be working at an intensity of 75 percent.

Take Charge of Your Health

To make it easy, you can use the following target heart rate training zone chart. In this chart, you see two numbers divided by a slash in each of the percentage columns. The first number is for the working heart rate. The second number is the number of heartbeats to count for ten seconds. You can use the second number if you don't want to do the multiplication to find your working heart rate.

TARGET HEART RATE TRAINING ZONE CHART			
Age	80%	70%	60%
15	164/27	144/24	123/21
16	163/27	143/24	122/21
17	162/27	142/24	122/21
18	162/27	141/24	121/20
19	161/27	141/24	121/20
20	160/27	140/23	120/20
21	159/27	139/23	119/20
22	158/26	139/23	119/20
23	158/26	138/23	118/20
24	157/26	137/23	118/20
25	156/26	137/23	117/20
26	155/26	136/23	116/19
27	154/26	135/23	116/19
28	154/26	134/22	115/19
29	153/26	134/22	115/19
30	152/25	133/22	114/19
31	151/25	132/22	113/19
32	150/25	132/22	113/19
33	150/25	131/22	112/19
34	149/25	130/22	119/19
35	148/25	130/22	119/19
36	147/25	129/22	110/18
37	146/24	128/21	110/18
38	146/24	127/21	109/18
39	145/24	127/21	109/18
40	144/24	126/21	108/18
41	143/24	125/21	107/18
42	142/24	124/41	107/18
43	142/24	124/21	106/18
44	141/24	123/21	106/18
45	140/23	123/21	105/18
46	139/23	122/20	104/17
47	138/23	121/20	104/17

48	138/23	120/20	103/17
49	137/23	120/20	103/17
50	136/23	119/20	102/17
51	135/23	118/20	101/17
52	134/22	118/20	101/17
53	134/22	117/20	100/17
54	133/22	116/19	100/17
55	132/22	116/19	99/17
56	131/22	115/19	98/16
57	130/22	114/19	98/16
58	130/22	113/19	97/16
59	129/22	113/19	97/16
60	128/21	112/19	93/16
61	127/21	111/19	95/16
62	126/21	111/19	95/16
63	126/21	110/18	94/16
64	125/21	109/18	94/16
65	124/21	108/18	93/16
66	123/21	108/18	92/15
67	122/20	107/18	92/15
68	122/20	106/18	91/15
69	121/20	106/18	91/15
70	120/20	105/18	90/15
71	119/20	104/17	89/15
72	118/20	104/17	89/15
73	118/20	103/17	88/15
74	117/20	102/17	88/15
75	116/19	102/17	87/15
76	115/19	101/17	86/14
77	114/19	100/17	86/14
78	114/19	99/17	85/14

Borg RPE Scale

Another way of assessing cardiorespiratory endurance is the rate of perceived exertion (RPE) method. It is valuable for determining intensity for several reasons, including helping clients to "listen to their bodies" and to anticipate approaching fatigue. The rate of perceived exertion can be used in conjunction with the heart rate method.

Using the original Borg scale of RPE, a rate of 12-13 approximates 50 percent of heart rate maximum and a rate of 16 approximates 85 percent of heart rate maximum. Therefore, it is recommended that you exercise within an RPE range of 12-16, meaning that the intensity feels somewhat hard to hard.

RPE (BORG) SCALE		
	6	No exertion at all
	7	Very, very light
	8	
	9	Very light
	10	
50%	11	Light
	12	
	13	Somewhat hard
	14	
	15	Hard
85%	16	
	17	Very hard
	18	
	19	Extremely hard
	20	Maximal exertion

Duration (Time)

It is recommended that a person exercise for twenty to sixty minutes continuously doing aerobic activity. This does not include warm-up and cooldown. Duration is inversely related to intensity: The lower the intensity, the longer the duration may be. For very de-conditioned people, several low-intensity, short-duration, ten-minute sessions may be more suitable.

Some examples of aerobic exercises are power walking, jogging, aerobic dancing, spinning, stair stepping, stationary cycling, indoor rowing, indoor cross-country skiing, jumping rope, outdoor cycling, outdoor rowing, swimming, and recreational sports.

How to Find Out How Cardiovascularly Fit You Are

It is very important to assess your current level of aerobic fitness so that you don't overdo or underdo your aerobic exercises. The step test is an easy way to calculate your cardiovascular fitness.

What You Need: A box or a step
              A stopwatch or a clock with a second hand
              Someone to help you time the test

What to Do: Start stepping up and down in a rhythmic motion on and
              off the step for a full three minutes. As soon as you're done,
              find your pulse and record the number of beats for one full

minute. You can also count your beats for ten seconds and multiply the number by six to get the total number of beats per minute. Check your fitness level in the following charts:

Norms for the Three-Minute Step Test (Men)			
	Age		
Fitness Category	18-25	26-35	36-45
Excellent	<79	<81	<83
Good	79-89	81-89	83-96
Above Average	90-99	90-99	97-103
Average	100-105	100-107	104-112
Below Average	106-116	108-117	113-119
Poor	117-128	118-128	120-130
Very Poor	>128	>128	>130
	Age		
Fitness Category	46-55	56-65	65+
Excellent	<87	<86	<88
Good	87-97	86-97	88-96
Above Average	98-105	98-103	97-103
Average	106-116	104-112	104-113
Below Average	117-122	113-120	114-120
Poor	123-132	121-129	121-130
Very Poor	>132	>129	>130

Norms for the Three-Minute Step Test (Women)			
	Age		
Fitness Category	18-25	26-35	36-45
Excellent	<85	<88	<90
Good	85-98	88-99	90-102
Above Average	99-108	100-111	103-110
Average	109-117	112-119	111-118
Below Average	118-126	120-126	119-128
Poor	127-140	127-138	129-140
Very Poor	>140	>138	>140
	Age		
Fitness Category	46-55	56-65	65+
Excellent	<94	<95	<90
Good	94-104	95-104	90-102
Above Average	105-115	105-112	103-115
Average	116-120	113-118	116-122
Below Average	121-126	119-128	123-128
Poor	127-135	129-139	129-134
Very Poor	>135	>139	>134

Muscular Strength and Endurance

The muscles in your body make up over 40 percent of your total body mass. Due to the large percentage of space they take up, they are responsible for a major portion of the energy reactions that take place in your body.

Metabolism is also known as energy consumption and is what is used to burn the calories we eat. Our metabolism will also burn stored energy in our bodies (fat) if it needs energy to do work and if it is not readily available. Muscle mass burns five times more calories than fat. The more muscle mass your body has, the higher your metabolism or energy burning capacity will be.

Several benefits of enhanced muscular strength and endurance:

- enhanced self-image
- injury prevention
- improved body composition
- improved performance of physical activities
- improved muscle and bone health with aging

Enhanced Self-Image

Weight training leads to an enhanced self-image by providing stronger, firmer-looking muscles and a toned, healthy-looking body. Men tend to build larger, stronger, more shapely muscles. Women tend to lose inches, increase strength, and develop greater muscle definition.

Because weight training provides measurable objectives (pounds lifted, repetitions accomplished), a person can easily recognize improved performance, leading to greater self-confidence.

Injury Prevention

Increased muscle strength provides protection against injury because it helps people maintain good posture and appropriate body mechanics when carrying out everyday activities like walking, lifting, and carrying. Strong muscles in the abdomen, hips, low back, and legs support the back in proper alignment and help prevent low-back pain, which afflicts over 85 percent of all Americans at some time in their lives. Training for muscular strength also makes the tendons, ligaments, and joint surfaces stronger and less susceptible to injury.

Improved Body Composition

Healthy body composition means that the body has a high proportion of fat-free mass (primarily composed of muscle) and a relatively small proportion of fat. Strength training improves body composition by increasing muscle mass, thereby tipping the body composition ratio toward fat-free mass and away from fat. Building muscle mass through strength training also helps with losing fat because metabolic rate is directly proportional to muscle mass: The more muscle mass, the higher the metabolic rate. A high metabolic rate means that a nutritionally sound diet will not lead to an increase in body fat.

Improved Performance of Physical Activities

A person with a moderate-to-high level of muscular strength and endurance can perform everyday tasks such as climbing stairs and carrying books or groceries with ease. Muscular strength and endurance are also important in recreational activities; people with poor muscle strength tire more easily and are less effective in activities like hiking, skiing, and playing tennis. Increased strength can enhance your enjoyment of recreational sports by making it possible to achieve high levels of performance and to handle advanced techniques.

Improved Muscle and Bone Health with Aging

Research has shown that good muscle strength helps people live healthier lives. A lifelong program of regular strength training prevents muscle and nerve degeneration that can compromise the quality of life and increase the risk of hip fractures and other potentially life-threatening injuries. After age thirty, people begin to lose muscle mass. As a person ages, motor nerves can become disconnected from the portion of muscle they control. Muscle physiologists estimate that by age seventy, 15 percent of the motor nerves in most people are no longer connected to muscle tissue. Aging and inactivity also cause muscles to become slower and therefore less able to perform quick, powerful movements. Strength training helps maintain motor-nerve connections and the quickness of muscles.

Osteoporosis is common in people over age fifty-five, particularly postmenopausal women. Osteoporosis leads to fractures that can be life threatening. Hormonal changes from aging account for much of the bone loss that occurs, but lack of bone stress due to inactivity and a poor diet are contributory factors. Recent research indicates that strength training can lessen bone loss even if it is taken up later in life. Increased muscle strength can also help prevent falls, which are a major cause of injury in people with osteoporosis.

What is Muscular Strength and Endurance?

Muscular strength and muscular endurance are distinct but related components of fitness. Muscular strength, the maximum amount of force a muscle can produce in a single effort, is usually assessed by measuring the maximum amount of weight a person can lift one time. This single maximal movement is referred to as one repetition maximum (1 RM).

Muscular endurance is the ability of a muscle to exert a submaximal force repeatedly or continuously overtime. This ability depends on muscular strength because a certain amount of strength is required for any muscle movement. Muscular endurance is usually assessed by counting the maximum number of repetitions of a muscular contraction a person can do. You can test the muscular endurance of a major muscle group in your body by taking the sixty-second-sit-up test or the curl-up test and the push-up test.

How Does Weight Training Work?

Muscles move the body and enable it to exert force because they move the skeleton. When a muscle contracts (shortens), it moves a bone by pulling on the tendon that attaches the muscle to the bone. Muscles consist of individual muscle cells, or muscle fibers, connected in bundles. A single muscle is made up of many bundles of muscle fibers and is covered by layers of connective tissue that hold the fibers together. Muscle fibers, in turn, are made up of smaller units called myofibrils. (When your muscles are given the signal to contract, protein filaments within the myofibrils slide across one another, causing the muscle fiber to shorten.) Weight training causes the size of individual muscle fibers to increase by increasing the number of myofibrils. Larger muscle fibers mean a larger and stronger muscle. The development of larger muscle fibers is called hypertrophy.

Muscle fibers are classified as fast-twitch or slow-twitch fibers according to their strength, speed of contraction, and energy source. Slow-twitch fibers are relatively fatigue resistant, but they don't contract as rapidly or strongly as fast-twitch fibers. The main energy system that fuels slow-twitch fibers is aerobic. Fast-twitch fibers contract more rapidly and forcefully than slow-twitch fibers but fatigue more quickly. Although oxygen is important in the energy system that fuels fast-twitch fibers, they rely more on anaerobic metabolism than slow-twitch fibers do.

Most muscles contain a mixture of slow-twitch and fast-twitch fibers. The type of fiber that acts depends on the type of work required. Endurance activities like jogging tend to use slow-twitch fibers, whereas strength and power activities like sprinting use fast-twitch fibers. Weight training can increase the size and strength of both fast-twitch and slow-twitch fibers, although fast-twitch fibers are mostly increased.

Types of Weight Training Exercises

Weight training exercises are generally classified as isometric or isotonic. Each involves a different way of using and strengthening muscles.

Isometric exercise, also called static exercise, involves applying force without movement. To perform an isometric exercise, a person can use an immovable object like a wall to provide resistance, or the individual can just tighten a muscle while remaining still (for example, tightening the abdominal muscles while sitting at a desk). In isometrics, the muscle contracts, but there is no movement.

Isometric exercises aren't as widely used as isotonic exercises because they don't develop strength throughout a joint's entire range of motion.

Isotonic (or dynamic) exercise involves applying force with movement. Isotonic exercises are the most popular type of exercises for increasing muscle strength and seem to be the most valuable for developing strength that can be transferred to other forms of physical activity. They can be performed with weight machines, free weights, or a person's own body weight (as in sit-ups or push-ups).

There are two kinds of isotonic muscle contractions: concentric and eccentric. A concentric muscle contraction occurs when the muscle applies force as it shortens. An eccentric muscle contraction occurs when the muscle applies force as it lengthens. For example, in an arm curl, the biceps muscle works concentrically as the weight is raised toward the shoulder and eccentrically as the weight is lowered.

Exercises

A complete weight training program works all the major muscle groups. It usually takes about eight to ten different exercises to get a complete workout. For overall fitness, you need to include exercises for your neck, upper back, shoulders, arms, chest, abdomen, lower back, thighs, buttocks, and calves.

The order of exercises can also be important. Do exercises for large muscle groups, or for more than one joint, before you do exercises that use small muscle groups or single joint. This allows for more effective overload of the larger, more powerful muscle groups. Small-muscle groups fatigue more easily than larger ones, and small-muscle fatigue limits your capacity to overload larger muscle groups. For example, lateral raises, which work the shoulder muscles, should be performed after bench presses, which work the chest and arms in addition to the shoulders. If you fatigue your shoulder muscles by doing lateral raises first, you won't be able to lift as much weight and effectively fatigue all the key muscle groups used during the bench press.

Resistance

The amount of weight (resistance) you lift in weight training exercises is equivalent in intensity to cardiorespiratory endurance training. It determines the way your body will adapt to weight training and how quickly these adaptations will occur. Choose weights based on your current level of muscular fitness and your fitness goals. To build strength rapidly, you should lift weights as heavy as 80 percent of your maximum capacity (1 RM). If you are more interested in building endurance, choose a lighter weight, perhaps 40-60 percent of 1 RM. For example, if your maximum capacity for the leg press is 160 pounds, you might lift 130 pounds to build strength and 80 pounds to build endurance. For a general fitness program to develop both strength and endurance, choose a weight in the middle of this range, perhaps 70 percent of 1 RM.

Because it can be time-consuming to continually reassess your maximum capacity for each exercise, you might find it easier to choose a weight based on the number of repetitions of an exercise you can perform with a given resistance. For example, find a weight that will allow your muscles to fatigue between eight and twelve repetitions.

Repetitions and Sets

In order to improve fitness, you must do enough repetitions of each exercise to fatigue your muscles. The number of repetitions needed to cause fatigue depends on the amount of resistance: The heavier the weight, the fewer repetitions to reach fatigue. In general, a heavyweight and a low number of repetitions (one to five) build strength, whereas a lightweight and a high number of repetitions (fifteen to twenty) build endurance. For a general fitness program to build both strength and endurance, try to do about eight to twelve repetitions of each exercise; a few exercises, such as abdominal crunches and calf raises, may require more. Choose a weight heavy enough to fatigue your muscles but light enough for you to complete the repetitions with good form. Due to an increased risk of injury, it is recommended that older and more frail people (approximately fifty to sixty years of age and above) perform more repetitions (ten to fifteen) using a lighter weight.

In weight training, a "set" refers to a group of repetitions of an exercise followed by a rest period. Surprisingly, exercise scientists have not identified the optimal number of sets for increasing strength. For developing strength and endurance for general fitness, a single set of each exercise is sufficient, provided you use enough resistance to fatigue your muscles. (You should just barely be able to complete the eight-to-twelve repetitions for each exercise.) Doing more than one set of each exercise may increase strength development, and most serious weight trainers do at least three sets of each exercise.

If you perform more than one set of an exercise, you need to rest long enough between sets to allow your muscles to work at a high-enough intensity to increase fitness. The length of the rest interval depends on the amount of resistance. In a program to develop a combination of strength and endurance for wellness, a rest period of one to three minutes between sets is appropriate. If you are lifting heavier loads to build maximum strength, rest three to five minutes between sets. You can save time in your workouts if you alternate sets of different exercises. Each muscle group can rest between sets while you work on other muscles.

Warm-up and Cooldown

As with cardiorespiratory endurance exercise, you should warm up before every weight training session and cool down afterward. You should do both a general warm-up—several minutes of walking or easy jogging—and a warm-up for the weight training exercises you plan to perform. For example, if you plan to do one or more sets of ten repetitions of bench presses with 125 pounds, you might do one set of ten repetitions with 50 pounds as a warm-up. Do similar warm-up exercises for each exercise in your program.

To cool down after weight training, relax for five to ten minutes after your workout. Including a period of postexercise stretching may help prevent muscle soreness. Warmed-up muscles and joints make this a particularly good time to work on flexibility.

Frequency of Exercise

For general fitness, the American College of Sports Medicine recommends a frequency of two to three days per week for weight training. Allow your muscles at least one day of rest between workouts. If you train too often, your muscles won't be able to work at a high-enough intensity to improve their fitness, and soreness and injury are more likely to result. If you enjoy weight training and would like to train more often, try working different muscle groups on alternate days. For example, work your arms and upper body one day, work your lower body the next day, and then return to upper body exercises on the third day.

A Sample Weight Training Program for General Fitness

Guidelines

Type of activity:	8-10 weight training exercises that focus on major muscle groups
Frequency:	2-3 days per week
Resistance:	Weights heavy enough to cause muscle fatigue when performed for the selected number of repetitions
Repetitions:	8-12 of each exercise (10-15 with a lower weight for people over age 50-60)
Sets:	1-3 (Doing more than one set per exercise may result in faster and greater strength gains.)

SAMPLE PROGRAM				
	Exercise	Resistance (10)	Repetitions	Sets
1	Bench Press	60	10	1-3
2	Overhead Press	40	10	1-3
3	Lat Pulls	40	10	1-3
4	Lateral Raises	10	10	1-3
5	Biceps Curls	25	10	1-3
6	Squats	30	10	1-3
7	Toe Raises	25	15	1-3
8	Abdominal Curls	—	30	1-3
9	Spine Extensions	—	10	1-3
10	Neck Flexion	—	10	1-3

The Weight Training Exercises

Exercise 1—Bench Press

Muscles Developed: Pectoralis major, triceps, deltoids

Instructions:

A. Lying on a bench on your back, with your feet on the floor, grasp the bar with palms upward and hands shoulder-width apart.

B. Lower the bar to your chest. Then return it to the starting position. The bar should follow an elliptical path, during which the weight moves from a low point at the chest to a high point over the chin. If your back arches too much, try doing this exercise with your feet on the bench.

Exercise 2—Overhead Press

Muscles Developed: Deltoids, triceps, trapezius

Instructions:

This exercise can be done standing or sitting with dumbbells or barbells. The shoulder press begins with the weight at your chest.

A.   Grasp the weight with your palms facing away from you.

B.   Push the weight overhead until your arms are extended (do not lock your elbows). Then return to the starting position (weight at chest). Be careful not to arch your back excessively.

Exercise 3—Lat Pulls

Muscles Developed: Latisimus dorsi, biceps

Instructions:

Begin in a seated or kneeling position, depending on the type of lat machine and the manufacturer's instructions.

A. Grasp the bar of the machine with arms fully extended.

B. Slowly pull the weight down until it reaches the back of your neck. Slowly return to the starting position.

Exercise 4—Lateral Raise

Muscles Developed: Deltoids

Instructions:

A. Stand with feet shoulder-width apart and a dumbbell in each hand. Hold the dumbbells parallel to each other.

B. With elbows slightly bent, slowly lift both weights until they reach shoulder level. Keep your wrists in a neutral position, in-line with your forearms. Return to the starting position.

Exercise 5—Biceps Curl

Muscles Developed: Biceps, brachialis

Instructions:

A. From a standing position, grasp the bar with your palms upward and your hands shoulder-width apart.

B. Keeping your upper body rigid, flex (bend) your elbows until the bar reaches a level slightly below the collarbone. Return the bar to the starting position.

Exercise 6—Squat

Muscles Developed: Quadriceps, gluteus maximus, hamstrings, gastrocnemius

Instructions:

Stand with feet shoulder-width apart and toes pointed slightly outward.

A. Rest the bar on the back of your shoulders, holding it there with hands facing forward.

B. Keeping your head up and lower back straight, squat down until your thighs are almost parallel with the floor. Drive upward toward the starting position, keeping your back in a fixed position throughout the exercise.

Exercise 7—Toe Raise

Muscles Developed: Gastrocnemius, soleus

Instructions:

Stand with feet shoulder-width apart and toes pointed straight ahcad.

A. Rest the bar on the back of your shoulders, holding it there with hands facing forward.

B. Press down with your toes while lifting your heels. Return to the starting position.

Exercise 8—Abdominal Curl

Muscles Developed: Rectus abdominis, obliques

Instructions:

A.   Lie on your back on the floor with your arms folded across your chest and your feet on the floor or a bench.

B.   Curl your trunk up and forward by raising your head and shoulders from the ground. Lower to the starting position.

Exercise 9—Spine Extensions

Muscles Developed: Erector spinae, gluteus maximus, hamstrings, deltoids

Instructions:

Begin on all fours with your knees below your hips and your hands below your shoulders.

Unilateral Spine Extension:

A.   Extend your right leg to the rear, and reach forward with your right arm. Keep your neck neutral and your raised arm and leg in-line with your torso. Don't arch your back or let your hip or shoulder sag. Hold this position for ten to thirty seconds. Repeat with your left leg and left arm.

Bilateral Spine Extension:

B.   Extend your left leg to the rear and reach forward with your right arm. Keep your neck neutral and your raised leg in-line with your torso. Don't arch your back or let your hip or shoulder sag. Hold this position for ten to thirty seconds. Repeat with your right leg and right arm.

Exercise 10—Neck Flexion and Lateral Flexion

Muscles Developed: Sternocleidomastoids, scaleni

Instructions:

Neck Flexion:

A. Place your hand on your forehead with fingertips pointed up. Using the muscles at the back of your neck, press your head forward and resist the pressure with the palm of your hand.

Lateral Flexion:

B. Place your hand on the right side of your face, fingertips pointed up. Using the muscles on the left side of your neck, press your head to the right and resist the pressure with the palm of your hand. Repeat on the left side.

Alternate Your Weight Training Days

If you find that you really enjoy weight training and would like to do it more than two to three days a week, alternate your workouts between upper body one day and lower body the next.

The following are exercises you will do on the day for your upper body workout:

Warm-Up

As always, begin with a five-minute aerobic warm-up to get your heart pumping and to get freshly oxygenated blood to your muscles. You can do this by marching in place, doing side steps, jogging in place, or a combination of all three.

A Few Simple Stretches

Deep Breath

1. Take a deep breath.

2. Inhale through the nose as your arms flow out to the sides and up overhead. Exhale out the mouth as your arms slowly come down to your sides.

3. Repeat three times.

Full-Body Stretch

This is a great stretch for your whole body, especially your arms, shoulders, and spine. You can do this one either sitting or standing.

1. Lift your arms above your head and reach as high as you can.

2. Make sure you breathe while holding this stretch for five to fifteen seconds.

3. Bring your arms down in front of you and relax.

Modification:

Side Stretch—Slowly bend slightly to the left and then to the right.

Triceps Stretch

Designed to stretch the muscles of the backs of your upper arms, it can be performed either sitting or standing. In addition to doing this one at the beginning and the end of your workout, you might find it beneficial to perform the stretch in between exercises.

1. Raise your right arm above you and bend the elbow so your right hand is behind your neck.

2. With your left hand, grasp your right elbow and gently pull the elbow behind your head.

3. Hold the stretch for fifteen to twenty seconds.

4. You should feel a nice stretch in your right triceps.

5. Relax and repeat the stretch on the left arm.

Your Upper Body Workout

Pec Press (with weights)

Muscles Worked: Chest (pectoralis)

Instructions:

1. Lie on your back with your knees bent and your feet on the floor.

2. With the weights in your hands, slowly bend your arms so that your elbows are parallel to your shoulders.

3. Push the weights straight up so that your arms are extended directly over your chest.

4. Return to starting position.

5. Repeat the movement.

Do three sets of eight-to-twelve reps each. Rest fifteen seconds between sets.

Chest Flys (with weights)

Muscles Worked: Chest (pectoralis)

Instructions:

1. Lie on your back on the floor with your knees bent and your feet flat on the floor.

2. Hold the weights in your hands with your arms extended straight-out at shoulder level, above your chest, with palms facing inward.

3. Slowly lower your arms to your side, keeping them bent at the same angle throughout the movement.

4. Slowly return your arms to the starting position by squeezing your chest as if you're making a cleavage and repeating the movement.

Do three sets of eight-to-twelve reps each. Rest fifteen seconds between sets.

Biceps Curl (with weights)

Muscles Worked: Biceps

Instructions:

1. Sit on the floor with your legs crossed in front of you. Your back should be straight and your abs tight.

2. With an underhand grip, hold the weights at your sides with your arms extended.

3. Exhale as you slowly raise the weights toward your upper arms and shoulders, bending your elbows.

4. Hold momentarily and return your hands to the starting position. Be sure that you keep your elbows close to your body throughout the movement.

Do three sets of eight-to-twelve reps each. Rest fifteen seconds between sets.

Lateral-Side Raises (with weights)

Muscles Worked: Shoulders (deltoids)

Instructions:

1. Stand with your feet shoulder-width apart, abs tight, back straight, and knees slightly bent.

2. Hold weights at your side.

3. Raise the weights out to your sides. Arms should be straight and palms down. Return to the starting position.

4. Continue to complete lateral-side raises up and down.

Do three sets of eight-to-twelve reps each. Rest fifteen seconds between sets.

Triceps Toner (with weights)

Muscles Worked: Back of arms (triceps)

Instructions:

1. Stand with your feet shoulder-width apart and knees slightly bent with weights in your hands. Keep your abs tight, back flat, and bend slightly forward at the waist.

2. Raise your elbows so that the upper part of your arms is parallel with the floor. Keep your elbows close to your body.

3. Straighten your arms. Be sure to squeeze your triceps as you do so.

4. Return your hands to the starting position, pause, and repeat the movement.

Do three sets of eight-to-twelve reps each. Rest fifteen seconds between sets.

The Chest Press

Muscles Worked: Chest and back of upper arms (pecs and triceps)

Instructions:

1. Lie with your back flat on a bench and with your knees bent. Keep your back flat against the bench with little or no arch. Hold the appropriate weight in each hand, slightly above chest level and with your palms facing forward.

2. Contract your abdominal muscles. Gradually raise both dumbbells up until your arms are fully extended above your chest. Do not lock your elbows. Slowly return the dumbbells back to the starting position. Control your movements throughout the entire exercise, exhaling when raising the dumbbells and inhaling on the return.

3. Keep your head and back firmly against the bench throughout the entire exercise.

Do three sets of eight-to-twelve reps each. Rest fifteen seconds between sets.

The Shoulder Press

Muscles Worked: Shoulders

Instructions:

1. Sit upright in a chair with your back supported and your feet flat on the floor. Keep your back flat against the back of the chair with little or no arch. Hold the appropriate weight in each hand, slightly above shoulder level and with your palms facing forward. Keep your elbows out to the side.

2. Contract your abdominal muscles. Keeping your palms facing forward, raise the weights up and inward until the inside ends of the dumbbells are nearly touching each other and are directly overhead. Do not lock your elbows. Pause, then lower the dumbbells slowly to the starting position. Control your movements throughout the entire exercise, exhaling upon raising the dumbbells and inhaling on the return.

Do three sets of eight-to-twelve reps each. Rest fifteen seconds between sets.

The Triceps Extension

Muscles Worked: Back of upper arms (triceps)

Instructions:

1. Stand straight with your feet slightly apart and your knees slightly bent. Using an interlocking grip, hold a dumbbell of the appropriate weight above your head with your arms fully extended.

2. Contract your abdominal muscles. Slowly lower the dumbbell back behind your head and neck while keeping your elbows in place above your head. Continue until your forearms are parallel to the floor.

3. Control your movements and maintain your posture throughout the entire exercise. Pause, then gradually raise the dumbbell back up to the starting position. Inhale while lowering the dumbbell down and exhale when raising it up.

Do three sets of eight-to-twelve reps each. Rest fifteen seconds between sets.

One-Arm Row (with weights)

Muscles Worked: Upper back (latisimus dorsi, rhomboid),
back of shoulders (posterior deltoid)

Instructions:

1.   Stand with your feet apart, left foot in front of the right.

2.   Bend your knees slightly, and keep your abs tight.

3.   Rest the palm of your left hand on your left thigh. Holding the weight in your right hand, let your arm extend to the floor.

4.   Pull the weight up to your armpit, then lower it back to the starting position and repeat.

Do three sets of eight-to-twelve reps each. Rest fifteen seconds between sets.

Push-Ups

Muscles Worked: Chest (pectoralis), shoulders (anterior deltoid), triceps

Instructions:

1. Kneel on the floor with your ankles crossed and your hands out in front of you on the floor.

2. Straighten your back, with abs tight and your head in a natural position.

3. Slowly bend your elbows, and lower your chest to the floor.

4. Straighten your elbows, and return to the starting position.

Do three sets of eight-to-twelve reps each. Rest fifteen seconds between sets.

Your Lower Body Workouts and Exercises

Warm-Up

As always, begin with a five-minute aerobic warm-up to get your heart pumping and to get freshly oxygenated blood to your muscles. You can do this by marching in place, doing side steps, jogging in place, or a combination of all three.

Next—A Few Simple Stretches

Quad Stretch

Your quadriceps is the four muscles in the front of your thighs. They are among the largest and strongest muscle groups in your body and are used in every activity.

1. Lie on your side with your legs together.

2. Bend your right leg behind you, and grasp the foot or the ankle.

3. Gently pull your foot toward your buttocks.

4. When you feel tension in the front of your thighs, hold the stretch fifteen to twenty seconds.

5. Switch sides and repeat the movement with the left leg.

Reach for Toes

This is a great stretch for the backs of your legs (hamstrings) and your lower back (erector spinae). Placing the towel under your buttocks will assist you in achieving proper form, making the exercise easier and more effective. The correct technique is to keep your back straight and to lengthen the space between your sternum and pelvic bone. Don't hunch shoulders forward.

1. Sit on the floor, place a towel under your buttocks, and keep your legs straight-out in front of you.

2. Sit up with your back straight, abs tight, and toes pointing to the ceiling.

3. Exhale as you bend forward, reaching your hands toward your toes.

4. Be sure that you keep your legs and back as straight as you possibly can.

5. Hold the stretch for fifteen to twenty seconds, relax, and repeat.

Hamstring Stretch

This is a wonderful stretch for the back of the legs (hamstrings). It is especially useful if your lower back is bothering you. As with the rest of your stretches, be sure to breathe, relax, and never bounce.

1. Lie on your back on the floor with your knees bent and your feet on the floor.

2. Raise your right leg up, and pull it toward your chest. You can use a towel to assist you.

3. Hold the stretch for fifteen to twenty seconds.

4. Lower the leg and repeat the stretch with the left leg.

Lower Body Exercises

Basic Stomach Crunch

Muscles Worked: Abdominals (rectus abdominis)

Instructions:

1. Lie on your back with your knees bent and your feet on the floor. (If you are a beginner, or have neck problems, use a pillow under your neck and head.)

2. Press your lower back firmly into the floor. There should be no arch in your back at all.

3. Rest your head in your hands, but keep your neck and shoulders relaxed.

4. Tighten your abdominals and slowly lift your shoulders up off the floor (about six inches).

5. Exhale as you crunch. Keep your elbows back and chin up as if you have an apple between your chin and chest.

6. Slowly lower your shoulders back to the floor and repeat.

Do three sets of eight-to-twelve crunches each. Rest fifteen seconds between sets.

Basic Squats

Muscles Worked: Thighs (quadriceps), buttocks (gluteals), hamstrings

Instructions:

1. Stand with your feet a little wider than your hips. Your back should be straight and your abs tight.

2. Place your hands on your hips.

3. Bend your knees and begin to squat. Feel as though you're sitting back, with your body weight through your heels. Hips should move behind your heels, like you are lowering yourself into a chair. Simultaneously raise your hands in front of you—this will help you balance.

4. As you stand back up, exhale and squeeze your buttocks. Repeat.

5. Never go lower than a ninety-degree angle.

Do three sets of eight-to-twelve crunches each. Rest fifteen seconds between sets.

Basic Outer Thigh Leg Lift

Muscles Worked: Outer thigh (abductors)

Instructions:

1. Lie on the floor with your left side down. Your head, shoulders, and hips should all be aligned.

2. Bend your left leg, putting your right hand down in front of you for balance.

3. Keeping your right leg straight and your foot flexed, slowly raise your leg. Lower it back to the floor, then repeat. This is a very short movement, so be careful not to raise your leg too high. You should be focusing on the outer thigh of your top leg.

Do three sets of eight-to-twelve leg lifts on each leg.

Basic Inner Thigh Lift

Muscles Worked: Inner thigh (adductors)

Instructions:

1. Lie on the floor on your left side. Your head, shoulders, and hips should all be aligned.

2. Bend your right leg and place it on the floor in front of you.

3. Slowly raise your left leg off the floor to a comfortable height. Try to keep it straight.

4. Pause at the top of the movement, then lower the leg back to the floor. Repeat.

5. Your left foot should remain flexed and parallel to the floor throughout the movement.

Do three sets of eight-to-twelve leg lifts on each leg.

Walking Lunges

Muscles Worked: Thighs (quadriceps), buttocks (gluteals), hamstrings

Instructions:

1. Hold weights at your sides (weights optional). Start with your feet about shoulder-width apart.

2. Take a step with one foot. As you take your step, bend your back knee toward the floor. Be sure you don't bang your knee on the floor. Your body weight should be on your front heel and on your back toes.

3. Rise back up, and as you do, bring your back foot forward to return to the starting position.

4. Take giant steps forward, alternating legs.

Do three sets of eight-to-twelve lunges each. Rest fifteen seconds between sets.

Calf Raises

Muscles Worked: Calves (gastrocnemius)

Instructions:

1. Stand with your feet together. Place your hands on the back of a chair for balance.

2. Raise up on your toes so that you are on the balls of your feet. As you rise, be sure to really squeeze your calves.

3. Lower your heels back to the floor and repeat. This exercise can also be done one leg at a time to make it a little tougher.

Do three sets of eight-to-twelve leg raises. Rest fifteen seconds between sets.

Oblique Crunch

Muscles Worked: Obliques

Instructions:

1. Lie on your back with knees bent and feet flat on the floor. Make sure the small of the back is pressed into the floor.

2. Contract the abdominals as you lift your head and shoulders about six inches from the floor.

3. Twist slightly to the side, reaching your hands to the outside of your right thigh. Hold the reach, and try to keep shoulders off the floor, pulsing (lifting up and down). Those of you who need support for your neck, place your hands behind your head. Your abdominal muscles should be contracted the entire time. Your goal is to keep the shoulder blades off the floor.

4. Hold the reach while pulsing. After completing three sets on the right side, repeat on the left side.

Do three sets of eight-to-twelve crunches each.

Upper Body Firmer (with weights)

Muscles Worked: Shoulders (posterior deltoid), upper back (rhomboids)

Instructions:

1. Sit in a chair. Lean forward so your chest is near your thighs.

2. With weights in your hands, slowly lift your arms straight-out to the sides, your pinkies up.

3. Squeeze your shoulder blades together. Return to the starting position and repeat the movement. Make sure that your movement is slow and deliberate; try not to swing the weights.

Do three sets of eight to twelve each.

Buttocks Firmer

Muscles Worked: Buttocks (gluteals)

Instructions:

1. Kneel on the floor with your elbows and hands on the floor.

2. Be sure to keep your back flat, abs tight, and your hips square to the floor.

3. Raise your right leg from the floor, keeping it bent at a right angle. Your upper leg and right foot should be parallel to the floor.

4. Slowly raise your knee up and down, pressing your foot toward the ceiling, squeezing your buttocks.

Do three sets of eight-to-twelve reps for each leg. Rest fifteen seconds between sets.

Power Lunge

Muscles Worked: Thighs (quadriceps), hamstrings, buttocks (gluteals)

Instructions:

1. Start with your feet about shoulder-width apart (weights optional).

2. Take a step forward with one foot. Make sure front knee stays at a ninety-degree angle. Keep your knee in a line with your ankle.

3. As you step forward, bend your back knee. Be sure you don't bang it on the floor. Your weight should be balanced between your back toes and your front heel.

4. Push back to the starting position bringing legs together, and repeat alternating your legs.

Do three sets of eight-to-twelve reps each. Rest fifteen seconds between sets.

Flexibility

Flexibility

Flexibility is the ability of a joint to move through its full range of motion—it's extremely important for general fitness and wellness. The smooth and easy performance of everyday and recreational activities is impossible if flexibility is poor.

Flexibility is a highly adaptable physical fitness component. It increases in response to a regular program of stretching exercises and decreases with inactivity. Flexibility is also specific; good flexibility in one joint does not necessarily mean good flexibility in another. Flexibility can be increased through stretching exercises for all major joints.

There are two basic types of flexibility: static and dynamic. Static flexibility refers to the ability to assume and maintain an extended position at one end or point in a joint's range of motion; it is what most people mean by the term "flexibility." Dynamic flexibility, unlike static flexibility, involves movement. It is the ability to move a joint quickly through its range of motion with little resistance.

Static flexibility depends on many factors, including the structure of a joint and the tightness of muscles, tendons, and ligaments that are attached to it. Dynamic flexibility is dependent on static flexibility; but it also involves such factors as strength, coordination, and resistance to movement. Dynamic flexibility can be important for both daily activities and sports. However, because static flexibility is easier to measure and better researched, most assessment tests and stretching programs target static flexibility.

Benefits of Flexibility and Stretching Exercises

Good flexibility provides benefits for the entire muscular and skeletal system; it may also prevent injuries and soreness and improve performance in sports and other activities.

Joint Health

Good flexibility is essential to good joint health. When the muscles and other tissues that support a joint are tight, the joint is subject to abnormal stresses that can cause joint deterioration. For example, tight thigh muscles cause excessive pressure on the kneecap, leading to pain in the knee joint. Tight shoulder muscles can compress sensitive soft tissues in the shoulder, leading to pain and disability in the joint. Poor joint flexibility can also cause abnormalities in joint lubrication, leading to deterioration of the sensitive cartilage cells lining the joint. Pain and further joint injury can result.

Improved flexibility can greatly improve your quality of life, particularly as you get older. Aging decreases the natural elasticity of muscles, tendons, and joints, resulting in stiffness. The problem is compounded if you have arthritis. Flexibility exercises improve the elasticity in your tissues, making it easier to move your body. When you're flexible, every activity becomes easier.

Reduction of Postexercise Muscle Soreness

Delayed onset muscle soreness occurring one to two days after exercise is thought to be caused by damage to the muscle fibers and supporting connective tissue. Some studies have shown that stretching after exercise decreases the degree of muscle soreness.

Relief of Aches and Pains

Flexibility exercises help relieve pain that develops from stress or prolonged sitting. Studying or working in one place for a long time can cause your muscles to become tense. Stretching helps relieve tension, so you can go back to work refreshed and effective.

Improved Body Position and Strength

Good flexibility lets a person assume more efficient body positions and exert force through a greater range of motion. For example, swimmers with more flexible shoulders have stronger strokes because they can pull their arms through the water in the optimal position. Flexible joints and muscles let you move more fluidly without constraint. Some studies also suggest that flexibility training enhances strength development.

Maintenance of Good Posture

Good flexibility also contributes to body symmetry and good posture. Bad postural habits can gradually change your body structures. Sitting in a slumped position, for example, can lead to tightness in the muscles in the front of your chest and overstretching and looseness in the upper spine, causing a rounding of the upper back. This condition, called kyphosis, is common in older people. It may be prevented by doing stretching exercises regularly.

Relaxation

Flexibility exercises are a great way to relax. Studies have shown that doing flexibility exercises reduces mental tension, slows your breathing rate, and reduces blood pressure.

Assessing Flexibility

Because flexibility is specific to each joint, there are no tests of general flexibility. The most commonly used flexibility test is the sit-and-reach test. This test rates the flexibility of the muscles in the lower back and hamstrings. Flexibility in these muscles may be important in preventing low-back pain.

Sit-and-Reach Test

Equipment: A flexibility box or measuring device. If you make your own measuring device, use two pieces of wood twelve inches high, attached at right angles to each other. Use a ruler or yardstick to measure the extent of reach. With the low numbers of the ruler toward the person being tested, set the six-inch mark of the ruler at the foot line of the box.

Preparation: Warm up your muscles with some low-intensity activity such as marching or jogging in place for five minutes.

Instructions:

1. Remove your shoes, and sit facing the flexibility box with your knees fully extended and your feet about four inches apart. Your feet should be flat against the box.

2. Reach as far forward as you can with palms down and one hand placed on top of the other. Hold the position of maximum reach for one to two seconds. Keep your knees locked at all times.

3. Repeat the stretch two times. Your score is the most distant point reached with the fingertips of both hands on the third trial, measured to the nearest quarter of an inch.

Rating Your Flexibility

Find your score in the table below to determine your flexibility rating.

Ratings for Sit-and-Reach Test (Men)					
Age	Very Poor	Poor	Moderate	High	Very High
15-19	below 5.25	5.25-6.75	7.00-8.75	9.00-10.75	above 10.75
20-29	below 5.50	5.50-7.00	7.25-8.75	9.00-11.00	above 11.00
30-39	below 4.75	4.75-6.50	6.75-8.50	8.75-10.25	above 10.25
40-49	below 2.75	2.75-5.00	5.25-6.75	7.00-10.25	above 9.25
50-59	below 2.00	2.00-5.00	5.25-6.50	6.75-9.25	above 9.25
60 and over	below 1.75	1.75-3.25	3.50-5.25	5.50-8.50	above 8.50

Ratings for Sit-and-Reach Test (Women)					
Age	Very Poor	Poor	Moderate	High	Very High
15-19	below 7.25	7.25-8.75	9.00-10.50	10.75-12.25	above 12.25
20-29	below 6.75	6.75-8.50	8.75-10.00	10.25-11.50	above 11.50
30-39	below 6.50	6.50-8.00	8.25-9.50	9.75-11.50	above 11.50
40-49	below 5.50	5.50-7.25	7.50-8.75	9.00-10.50	above 10.50
50-59	below 5.50	5.50-7.25	7.50-8.50	8.75-10.75	above 10.75
60 and over	below 4.75	4.75-6.00	6.25-7.75	8.00-9.25	above 9.25

Intensity and Duration of Flexibility Exercises

For each exercise, slowly apply stretch to your muscles to the point of slight tension or mild discomfort. Hold the stretch for ten to thirty seconds. As you hold the stretch, the feeling of slight tension should slowly subside. At that point, try to stretch a bit farther. Throughout the stretch, try to relax and breathe easily. Rest for about thirty to sixty seconds between each stretch, and do at least four repetitions of each stretch.

Frequency of Flexibility Training

The American College of Sports Medicine recommends that stretching exercises be performed a minimum of two to three days per week. Many people do flexibility training more often—three to five days per week—for even greater benefits. It's best to stretch when your muscles are warm, so try incorporating stretching into your cooldown after cardiorespiratory-endurance exercise or weight training. Stretching can also be a part of your warm-up, but it's best to increase the temperature of your muscles first by doing a five-minute warm-up of marching or jogging in place.

Flexibility Exercises

Head Turns and Tilts

Areas Stretched: Neck, upper back

Instructions:

Head Turns: Turn your head to the right and hold the stretch. Repeat to the left.

Head Tilts: Tilt your head to the left and hold the stretch. Repeat to the right.

Variation: Place your right palm on your right cheek. Try to turn your head to the right as you resist with your hand. Repeat on the left side.

Across-the-Body Stretch

Areas Stretched: Shoulders, upper back

Instructions:

Keeping your back straight, cross your left arm in front of your body and grasp it with your right hand. Stretch your arm, shoulders, and back by gently pulling your arm as close to your body as possible. Repeat the stretch with your right arm.

Variation: Bend your right arm over and behind your head. Grasp your right hand with your left, and gently pull your arm until you feel the stretch. Repeat for your left arm.

Upper-Back Stretch

Areas Stretched: Upper back

Instructions:

Stand with your feet shoulder-width apart, knees slightly bent, and pelvis tucked under. Clasp your hands in front of your body, and press your palms forward.

Variation: In the same position, wrap your arms around your body as if you were giving yourself a hug.

Lateral Stretch

Areas Stretched: Trunk muscles

Instructions:

Stand with your feet shoulder-width apart, knees slightly bent, and pelvis tucked under. Raise one arm over your head and bend sideways from the waist. Support your trunk by placing the hand or forearm of your other arm on your thigh or hip for support. Be sure you bend directly sideways and don't move your body below the waist. Repeat on the other side.

Forward Lunge

Areas Stretched: Hip, front of thigh (quadriceps)

Instructions:

Step forward and flex your forward knee, keeping your knee directly above your ankle. Stretch your other leg back so that it is parallel to the floor. Press your hips forward and down to stretch. Your arms can be at your sides, on top of your knee, or on the ground for balance. Repeat on the other side.

Side Lunge

Areas Stretched: Inner thigh, hip, calf

Instructions:

Stand in a wide straddle with your legs turned out from your hip joints and your hands on your thighs. Lunge to one side by bending one knee and keeping the other leg straight. Keep your knee directly over your ankle; do not bend it more than ninety degrees. Repeat on the other side.

Trunk Rotation

Areas Stretched: Trunk, outer thigh and hip, lower back

Instructions:

Sit with your right leg straight, left leg bent and crossed over the right knee, and left hand on the floor next to your left hip. Turn your trunk as far as possible to the left by pushing against your left leg with your right forearm or elbow. Keep your left foot on the floor. Repeat on the other side.

Alternate Leg Stretch

Areas Stretched: Back of the thigh (hamstring), hip, knee, ankle, buttocks

Instructions:

Lie flat on your back with both legs straight.

    A.   Grasp your left leg behind the thigh and pull into your chest.

    B.   Hold this position and then extend your left leg toward the ceiling.

    C.   Hold this position, and then bring your left knee back to your chest and pull your toes toward your shin with your left hand. Stretch the back of the leg by attempting to straighten your knee.

Repeat for the other leg.

Modified Hurdler Stretch

Areas Stretched: Back of the thigh (hamstring), lower back

Instructions:

Sit with your right leg straight and your left leg tucked close to your body. Reach toward your right foot as far as possible. Repeat for the other leg.

Variation: As you stretch forward, alternately flex and point the foot of your extended leg.

Lower Leg Stretch

Areas Stretched: Back of the lower leg (calf, soleus, Achilles tendon)

Instructions:

Stand with one foot about one to two feet in front of the other, with both feet pointing forward.

A.   Keeping your back leg straight, lunge forward by bending your front knee and pushing your rear heel backward. Hold this position.

B.   Then pull your back foot in slightly, and bend your back knee. Shift your weight to your back leg. Hold.

Repeat on the other side.

Nutrition

Nutrition

Nutrition is a major component to health. What you eat affects your energy levels, well-being, and overall fitness. Eating habits can also be closely linked with certain diseases, disabling conditions, and other health problems. Of particular concern is the connection between lifetime nutritional habits and the risk of the major chronic diseases, including heart disease, cancer, stroke, and diabetes. On the more positive side, however, a well-planned diet in conjunction with a fitness program can help prevent such conditions and even reverse some of them.

Creating a diet plan to support maximum fitness and protect against disease is a two-part project. First, you have to know which nutrients are necessary and in what amounts. Second, you have to translate those requirements into a diet consisting of foods you like to eat that are both available and affordable. Once you have an idea of what constitutes a healthy diet for you, you may also have to make adjustments in your current diet to bring it into line with your goals.

Yes, food is delicious, but what is important for your health are the nutrients contained in those foods. Your body requires proteins, fats, carbohydrates, vitamins, minerals, and water—about forty-five essential nutrients. The word "essential" means that you must get these substances from food because your body is unable to manufacture them at all, or at least not fast enough to meet your physiological needs.

Nutrients are released into the body by the process of digestion, which breaks them down into compounds that the gastrointestinal tract can absorb and the body can use. In this form, the essential nutrients provide energy, build and maintain body tissues and regular body functions. There are six classes of essential nutrients—proteins, carbohydrates, fats, vitamins, minerals, and water.

Three of the six classes of nutrients supply energy: proteins, carbohydrates, and fats. Fats provide the most energy: nine calories per gram. Protein and carbohydrates each provide four calories per gram. Experts advise against high fat consumption, in part because fats provide so many calories. Given the typical American diet, most Americans do not need the extra calories to meet energy needs.

Meeting our energy needs is only one of the functions of food. All the nutrients perform other numerous vital functions. In terms of quantity, water is the most significant nutrient. The body is approximately 60 percent water and can survive only a few days without it. Vitamins and minerals are needed in much smaller quantities, but they are still vital.

Proteins

Protein is an important component of muscle, bone, blood, enzymes, cell membranes, and some hormones. Protein can also provide energy at four calories per gram of protein weight. Proteins are composed of amino acids. Twenty common amino acids are found in food; nine of these are essential to an adult diet: histidine, isoleucine, leucine, lysine, methionine, phenylalanine, threonine, tryptophan, and valine. "Essential" means that they are required for normal health and growth but must be provided in the diet because the body manufactures them in insufficient quantities, if at all. The other eleven amino acids can be produced by the body as long as the necessary ingredients are supplied by foods.

Foods are rated as "complete" protein sources if they supply all nine essential amino acids in adequate amounts. They are classified as "incomplete" protein sources if they supply only some. Meat, fish, poultry, eggs, milk, cheese, and other foods from animal sources provide complete proteins. Incomplete proteins come from plant sources such as beans, peas, and nuts. These are good sources of most essential amino acids but are usually low in one or two. Different vegetable proteins are low in different amino acids, so combinations can provide complete proteins. Vegetarians who eat no foods from animal sources can obtain all essential amino acids by eating a wide variety of foods each day.

Fats

At nine calories per gram, fats (also known as lipids) are the most concentrated source of energy. The fats stored in your body represent usable energy, help insulate your body, and support and cushion your organs. Fats in the diet help your body absorb fat-soluble vitamins and add important flavor and texture to foods. During periods of rest and light activity, fats are the major body fuel. The nervous system, brain, and red blood cells are fueled by carbohydrates; but most of the rest of the body's organs are fueled by fats. Two fats—linoleic acid and alpha-linolenic acid—are essential to the diet. They are key regulators of such body functions as the maintenance of blood pressure and the progress of a healthy pregnancy.

Types and Sources of Fats

Most of the fats in food and in your body are in the form of triglycerides, which are composed of a glycerine molecule plus three fatty acids. A fatty acid is made up of a chain of carbon atoms with oxygen attached at the end and hydrogen atoms attached along the length of the chain. Fatty acids differ in the length of their carbon atom chains and in their degree of saturation (the number of hydrogens attached to the chain). If every available band from each carbon atom in a fatty acid chain is attached to a hydrogen atom, the fatty acid is said to be saturated. If not all the available bands are taken up by hydrogens, the carbon atoms in the chain will form double bands with each other. Such fatty acids are called unsaturated fats. If there is only one double band, the fatty acid is call monounsaturated. If there are two or more double bands, the fatty acid is called polyunsaturated. The essential fatty acids—linoleic and alpha-linolenic acids—are both polyunsaturated.

Food fats are often composed of both saturated and unsaturated fatty acids. The dominant type of fatty acid determines the fat's characteristics. Food fats containing large amounts of saturated fatty acids are usually solid at room temperature (these are called "fats"). They are generally found in animal products. The leading sources of saturated fat in the American diet are unprocessed animal flesh (hamburgers, steaks, roasts), whole milk, cheese, hot dogs, and lunch meats. Food fats containing large amounts of monounsaturated and polyunsaturated fatty acids are usually from plant sources and are liquid at room temperature (these are called "oils"). Olive, canola, and peanut oils contain mostly monounsaturated fatty acids. Sunflower, corn, and safflower oils contain mostly polyunsaturated fatty acids.

There are exceptions to these generalizations. When unsaturated vegetable oils undergo the process of hydrogenation, a mixture of saturated and unsaturated fatty acids is produced. Hydrogenation turns many of the double bands in unsaturated fatty acids into single bands, increasing the degree of saturation and producing a more solid fat from a liquid oil. Hydrogenation also produces trans fatty acids, unsaturated fatty acids with an atypical shape that affects their behavior during cooking and in the body. Food manufacturers use hydrogenation to increase the stability of an oil so it can be reused for deep frying—to improve the texture of certain foods, to keep oil from separating out of peanut butter, and to extend the shelf life of foods made with oil. Hydrogenation is the process used to transform a liquid oil into margarine or vegetable shortening.

Many baked and fried foods are prepared with hydrogenated vegetable oils, so they can be relatively high in saturated and trans fatty acids. Leading sources of trans fatty acids in the American diet are deep-fried; fast-foods such as french fries and fried chicken or fish; baked and snack foods such as cakes, cookies, pastries, doughnuts, and chips; and stick margarine. In general, the more solid a hydrogenated oil is, the more saturated and trans fats it contains. For example, stick margarine typically contains more saturated and trans fatty acids than tub or squeeze margarine does. Smaller amounts of trans fats are found naturally in meat and milk.

Hydrogenated vegetable oils are not the only plant fats that contain saturated fats. Palm and coconut oils, although derived from plants, are also highly saturated. On the other hand, fish oils, derived from an animal source, are rich in polyunsaturated fats.

Recommended Fat Intake

You need only about one tablespoon (fifteen grams) of vegetable oil per day incorporated into your diet to supply the essential fats. The average American diet supplies considerably more than this amount. In fact, fats make up about 33 percent of our caloric intake. (This is the equivalent of about seventy-five grams or five tablespoons of fat per day.) Health experts recommended that we reduce our fat intake to 30 percent, but not less than 10 percent of total daily calories, with less than 10 percent coming from saturated fat.

Fats and Your Health

Different types of fats have very different effects on health. Many studies have examined the effects of dietary fat intake on blood cholesterol levels and the risk of heart disease. Saturated and trans fatty acids have been found to raise blood levels of low-density lipoprotein (LDL), or "bad" cholesterol, thereby increasing a person's risk of heart disease. Unsaturated fatty acids, on the other hand, lower LDL and may increase levels of high-density lipoprotein (HDL), or "good" cholesterol. To reduce the risk of heart disease, it is important to substitute unsaturated fats for saturated and trans fats.

Most Americans consume more saturated fat (11 percent of total calories) than trans fat (2-4 percent of total calories). The best way to reduce saturated fat in your diet is to lower your intake of meat and full-fat dairy products (whole milk, cream, butter, cheese, ice cream). To lower trans fats, decrease your intake of deep-fried foods and baked goods made with hydrogenated vegetable oils; use liquid oils rather than margarine. (Remember, the softer or more liquid a fat is, the less saturated and trans fat it is likely to contain.) Saturated fats are listed on the nutrition label of prepared foods. Trans fats are not, but you can check for the presence of hydrogenated oils on the ingredient list. If "partially hydrogenated" oils or fats or "vegetable shortening" appear near the top of the list, the product may be high in trans fats.

Research has indicated that certain forms of polyunsaturated fatty acids—known as omega-3 fatty acids and found in fish—may have a particularly positive effect on cardiovascular health. If the endmost double bands of a polyunsaturated fat occur, three carbons from the end of the fatty acid chain, an omega-3 form is produced. If the endmost double bands occur at the sixth carbon atom, an omega-6 form is produced. Most of the polyunsaturated fats currently consumed by Americans are omega-6 forms, primarily from corn oil and soybean oil. However, the consumption of omega-3 fatty acids in fish has been shown to reduce the tendency of blood to clot, to decrease inflammatory responses in the body, and to raise levels of HDL. It even appears to lower the risk of heart disease in some people. Because of these benefits, nutritionists now recommend that Americans increase the proportion of omega-3 polyunsaturated fats in their diet by increasing their consumption of fish to two or more times a week. Mackerel, herring, salmon, sardines, anchovies, tuna, and trout are all good sources of omega-3 fatty acids.

Dietary fat can affect health in other ways. Diets high in fat are associated with an increased risk of certain forms of cancer, especially colon cancer. A high-fat diet can also make weight management more difficult. Because fat is a concentrated source of calories (nine calories per gram versus four calories per gram for protein and carbohydrate), a high-fat diet is often a high-calorie diet that can lead to weight gain. In addition, there is some evidence that calories from fat are more easily converted to body fat than calories from protein or carbohydrate.

Although more research is needed on the precise effects of different types and amounts of fat on overall health, a great deal of evidence points to the fact that most people benefit from lowering their overall fat intake to recommended levels and substituting unsaturated fats for saturated and trans fats.

Carbohydrates

Carbohydrates function primarily to supply energy to body cells. Some cells, such as those in the brain and other parts of the nervous system and in the blood, use only carbohydrates for fuel. During high-intensity exercise, muscles also get most of their energy from carbohydrates. When we don't eat enough carbohydrates to satisfy the needs of the brain and red blood cells, our bodies synthesize carbohydrates from proteins. In situations of extreme deprivation, when the diet lacks sufficient amounts of both carbohydrates and proteins, the body turns to its own proteins, resulting in severe muscle wasting. This rarely occurs, however, because the body's daily carbohydrate requirement is filled by just three or four slices of bread.

Simple and Complex Carbohydrates

Carbohydrates are classified into two groups: simple and complex. Simple carbohydrates contain only one—or two-sugar units in each molecule. A one-sugar carbohydrate is called a monosaccharide; a two-sugar carbohydrate, a disaccharide. Simple carbohydrates include sucrose (table sugar), fructose (fruit sugar, honey), maltose (malt sugar), and lactose (milk sugar). They provide much of the sweetness in foods. Simple carbohydrates are found naturally in fruits and milk and are added to soft drinks, fruit drinks, candy, and sweet desserts.

Starches and most types of dietary fiber are complex carbohydrates. They consist of chains of many sugar molecules and are called polysaccharides. Starches are found in a variety of plants, especially grains (wheat, rye, rice, oats, barley, legumes, and tubers—potatoes and yams). Most other vegetables contain a mix of starches and simple carbohydrates. Dietary fiber is found in fruits, vegetables, and grains.

Many nutritionists also distinguish between refined (processed) and unrefined carbohydrates. The refinement of wheat flour, rice, and cereal grains transforms whole wheat flour to white flour, brown rice to white rice, and so on. Refined carbohydrates usually retain all the calories of their unrefined counterparts, but they tend to be much lower in fiber, vitamins, and minerals. In general, unrefined carbohydrates tend to take longer to chew and digest than refined ones. They also enter the bloodstream more slowly. This slower digestive pace tends to make people feel full sooner and for a longer period, lessening the chance that they will overeat and gain weight. It also helps keep blood sugar and insulin levels low, which may decrease the risk of diabetes and heart disease. For all these reasons, unrefined carbohydrates are recommended over those that have been refined.

During digestion in the mouth and small intestine, the body breaks down starches and disaccharides into monosaccharides, such as glucose, for absorption into the bloodstream. Once the glucose is absorbed, cells take it up and use it for energy. The liver and muscles also take up glucose and store it in the form of a starch called glycogen. The muscles use glycogen as fuel during endurance events or long workouts. Carbohydrates consumed in excess of the body's energy needs are changed into fat and stored. Whenever caloric intake exceeds caloric expenditure, fat storage can lead to weight gain. This is true whether the excess calories come from carbohydrates, proteins, or fats.

How Much Carbohydrate Should You Eat?

On the average, Americans consume over 250 grams of carbohydrates per day, well above the minimum of 50-100 grams of essential carbohydrate required by the body. However, health experts recommend that Americans increase their consumption of carbohydrates—particularly complex carbohydrates—to 55 percent of total daily calories.

Experts also recommend that Americans alter the proportion of simple and complex carbohydrates in the diet, lowering simple carbohydrate intake from 25 percent to 15 percent or less of total daily calories. To accomplish this change, reduce your intake of foods like candy, sweet desserts, soft drinks, and sweetened fruit drinks, which are high in simple sugars but low in other nutrients. The bulk of the simple carbohydrates in your diet should come from fruits, which are excellent sources of vitamins and minerals, and milk, which is high in protein and calcium. Instead of prepared foods high in added sugars, choose a variety of foods rich in complex, unrefined carbohydrates.

Fiber

Dietary fiber consists of carbohydrate plant substances that are difficult or impossible for humans to digest. Instead, fiber passes through the intestinal tract and provides bulk for feces in the large intestine, which in turn facilitates elimination. In the large intestine, some types of fiber are broken down by bacteria into acids and gases, which explain why consuming too much fiber can lead to intestinal gas. Because humans cannot digest dietary fiber, fiber is not a source of carbohydrate in the diet. However, the consumption of dietary fiber is necessary for good health.

Nutritionists classify dietary fiber as soluble or insoluble. Soluble fiber slows the body's absorption of glucose and binds cholesterol-containing compounds in the intestine, lowering blood cholesterol levels and reducing the risk of cardiovascular disease. Insoluble fiber binds water, making the feces bulkier and softer so they pass more easily and quickly through the intestines.

Both kinds of fiber contribute to disease prevention. A diet high in soluble fiber can help people manage diabetes and high blood cholesterol levels. A diet high in insoluble fiber can help prevent a variety of health problems, including constipation, hemorrhoids, and diverticulitis (a painful condition in which abnormal pouches form and become inflamed in the wall of the large intestine). Some studies have linked high levels of insoluble fiber in the diet with a decreased incidence of colon and rectal cancer; conversely, a low-fiber diet may increase the risk of colon cancer. There is even some evidence that high levels of insoluble fiber can suppress and reverse precancerous changes that can lead to colon and rectal cancer.

All plant foods contain some dietary fiber; but fruits, legumes, oats (especially oat bran), barley, and psyllium (found in some laxatives) are particularly rich in it. Wheat (especially wheat bran), cereals, grains, and vegetables are all good sources of insoluble fiber. However, the processing of packaged foods can remove fiber, so it's important to depend on fresh fruits and vegetables and foods made from whole (unrefined) grains as sources of dietary fiber.

Most experts believe the average person would benefit from an increase in daily fiber intake. Currently, most people consume about 15 grams of fiber a day, whereas the recommended daily amount is 20-35 grams of food fiber—not from supplements, which should be taken only under medical supervision. However, too much fiber—more than 40-60 grams a day—can cause health problems such as overlarge stools or the malabsorption of important minerals. In fiber intake, as in all aspects of nutrition, balance and moderation are key principles.

To increase the amount of fiber in your diet, try the following:

- Choose whole grain bread instead of white bread, brown rice instead of white rice, and whole wheat pasta instead of regular pasta.
- Select high-fiber breakfast cereals. Look for breads, crackers, and cereals that list a whole grain first in the ingredient list: whole wheat flour, whole grain oats, and whole grain rice are whole grains. White flour is not.
- Eat whole fruits rather than drinking fruit juice. Top cereals, yogurts, and desserts with berries, apple slices, or other fruits.
- Include beans in soups and salads. Prepare salads that combine raw vegetables with pasta, rice, or beans.
- Substitute bean dip for cheese-based or sour cream-based dips or spreads. Use raw vegetables rather than chips for dipping.

Vitamins

Vitamins are organic (carbon-containing) substances required in very small amounts to promote specific chemical reactions within living cells. Humans need thirteen vitamins. Four are fat soluble (A, D, E, and K); and nine are water soluble (C); and the eight B-complex vitamins: thiamin, riboflavin, niacin, vitamin B-6, folate, vitamin B-12, biotin, and pantothenic acid. Solubility affects how a vitamin is absorbed, transported, and stored in the body. The water-soluble vitamins are absorbed directly into the bloodstream where they travel freely. Excess water-soluble vitamins are detected by the kidneys and excreted in urine. Fat-soluble vitamins require a more complex digestive process; they are usually carried in the blood by special proteins and are stored in the body in fat tissues rather than excreted.

Vitamins and Their Functions

Vitamins help chemical reactions take place. They provide no energy to the body directly but help unleash the energy stored in carbohydrates, proteins, and fats. Vitamins are critical in the production of red blood cells and the maintenance of the nervous, skeletal, and immune systems. Some vitamins also form substances that act as antioxidants, which help preserve healthy cells in the body. Key vitamin antioxidants include vitamin E, vitamin C, and the vitamin A derivative beta-carotene.

Sources of Vitamins

The human body does not manufacture most of the vitamins it requires and must obtain them from foods. Vitamins are abundant in fruits, vegetables, and grains. In addition, many processed foods, such as flour and breakfast cereals, are enriched with certain vitamins during the manufacturing process. On the other hand, both vitamins and minerals can be lost or destroyed during the storage and cooking of foods.

A few vitamins are made in certain parts of the body: the skin makes vitamin D when it is exposed to sunlight, and intestinal bacteria make biotin and vitamin K.

Minerals

Minerals are inorganic (noncarbon-containing) compounds you need in relatively small amounts to help regulate body functions, aid in the growth and maintenance of body tissues, and help release energy. There are about seventeen essential minerals. The major minerals—those that the body needs in amounts exceeding one hundred milligrams—include calcium, phosphorus, magnesium, sodium, potassium, and chloride. The essential trace minerals—those that you need in minute amounts—include copper, fluoride, iodine, iron, selenium, and zinc.

Characteristic symptoms develop if an essential mineral is consumed in a quantity too small or too large for good health. The minerals most commonly lacking in the American diet are iron, calcium, zinc, and magnesium. Lean meats are rich in iron and zinc, while low-fat or nonfat dairy products are excellent sources for calcium. Plant foods are good sources of magnesium. Iron-deficiency anemia is a problem in some age groups, and researchers agree that poor calcium intakes are laying the foundation for future osteoporosis, especially in women.

Drink Up! (Water)

Water is the major component in both foods and the human body: You are composed of about 60 percent water. Your need for other nutrients, in terms of weight, is much less than your need for water. You can live up to fifty days without food, but only a few days without water.

Water is distributed all over the body, among lean and other tissues and in urine and other body fluids. Water is used in the digestion and absorption of food and is the medium in which most of the chemical reactions take place within the body. Some water-based fluids like blood transport substances around the body, while other fluids serve as lubricants or cushions. Water also helps regulate body temperature.

Water is contained in almost all foods, particularly in liquids, fruits, and vegetables. The foods and fluids you consume provide 80-90 percent of your daily water intake; the remainder is generated through metabolism. You lose water each day in urine, feces, and sweat and through evaporation in your lungs. To maintain a balance between water consumed and water lost, you need to take in about one milliliter of water for each calorie you burn—about two liters (or eight cups) of fluid per day, more if you live in a hot climate or engage in vigorous exercise.

147

Thirst is one of the body's first signs of dehydration that we can actually recognize. However, by the time we are actually thirsty, our cells have been needing fluid for quite some time. So drink before you are thirsty. Keep a record of how much water you drink a day. Remember, you need eight, eight-ounce glasses—so drink up!

Amazing Antioxidants

When the body uses oxygen or breaks down certain fats as a normal part of metabolism, it gives rise to substances called free radicals. Environmental factors such as cigarette smoke, exhaust fumes, radiation, excessive sunlight, certain drugs, and stress can increase free radical production. A free radical is a chemically unstable molecule that is missing an electron; it will react with any molecule it encounters from which it can take an electron. In their search for electrons, free radicals react with fats, proteins, and DNA, damaging cell membranes and mutating genes. Because of this, free radicals have been implicated in aging, cancer, cardiovascular disease, and degenerative diseases like arthritis.

Antioxidants found in foods can help rid the body of free radicals, thereby protecting cells. Antioxidants react with free radicals and donate electrons, rendering them harmless. Some antioxidants—such as vitamin C, vitamin E, and selenium—are also essential nutrients. Others, such as flavonoids found in citrus fruits, are not. Obtaining a regular intake of these nutrients is vital for maintaining health. Many fruits and vegetables are rich in antioxidants.

Fantastic Phytochemicals

Antioxidants are a particular type of phytochemical, a substance found in plant foods that may help prevent chronic disease. Researchers have just begun to identify and study all the different compounds found in foods, and many preliminary findings are promising. For example, certain proteins found in soy foods may help lower cholesterol levels. Sulforaphane, a compound isolated from broccoli and other cruciferous vegetables, may render some carcinogenic compounds harmless. Allyl sulfides, a group of chemicals found in garlic and onions, appear to boost the activity of cancer-fighting immune cells. Further research on phytochemicals may extend the role of nutrition to the prevention and treatment of many chronic diseases.

If you want to increase your intake of phytochemicals, it is best to obtain them by eating a variety of fruits and vegetables rather than relying on supplements. It is likely that their health benefits are the result of chemical substances working in combination. Like many vitamins and minerals, isolated phytochemicals may be harmful if taken in high doses, so eat a variety of foods and enjoy all the benefits that phytochemicals have to offer.

Your Thirty-Day Fitness Program

At this point, you have gathered all the information on healthy eating, exercise, and how both contribute to preventing disease. Now it's time to take action.

If losing weight is one of your goals (and it is for most of us), you need to create a negative caloric balance. Taking off pounds is a mathematical equation. You must take in lesser calories than you burn off in a given day. One pound is equal to 3,500 calories. Losing weight properly should be consistent at about one to two pounds per week. I suggest that your goal be one pound a week.

Complete the following calculations to determine your weekly and daily negative caloric balance goals and the number of weeks to achieve your target weight.

Current weight: _____ lb.

Minus target weight: _____ lb.

Total weight to lose:_____ lb.

Total weight to lose (_____ lb.) ÷ weight to lose each week (_____ lb.)

= time to achieve target weight: _____ weeks

Weight to lose each week (_____ lb.) x 3,500 calories

= weekly negative caloric balance (cal/week)

Weekly negative caloric balance (_____ cal/week) ÷ 7 days/week

= daily negative caloric balance or _____ cal/day

Remember: keep your weight loss program on schedule. You must achieve the daily negative caloric balance by either decreasing your caloric consumption (eating less) or increasing your caloric expenditure (being more active). A combination of the two strategies will probably be most successful.

You can use the above calculation if your weight loss goal is more than one pound a week. If losing one pound a week feels right to you, then you can figure on decreasing your caloric intake by five hundred calories a day.

The following will be a thirty-day exercise and nutrition log so that you can see your progress on paper. It would be extremely helpful to get a pocket-sized calorie-counting book. If you do not want to do this, just read the label on the side of the food item. It is important to become acquainted with "serving sizes." You may want to use a small scale until you become familiar with what a size looks like.

Most people need a two-thousand-calorie diet to maintain their current weight. So we will use this as our starting point. If you find that you are losing weight too quickly (or slowly), you can adjust this number a couple of hundred calories in either direction.

Remember, when making food choices, your best bet is to incorporate lots of fruits and vegetables, whole grains, and lean meats. Oh, and don't forget your eight eight-ounce glasses of water every day. Congratulations on a new and healthy you, and good luck!

Day 1

Breakfast	Calories _____
Snack	Calories _____
Lunch	Calories _____
Dinner	Calories _____
Snack	Calories _____

Total calories for the day   Calories _____

Total number of eight-ounce glasses of water   _____
(minimum of eight glasses)

Total number of minutes of aerobic exercise   _____
(minimum of twenty minutes)

Weight training program for general fitness. Eight-to-ten weight training exercises that focus on major muscle groups done two to three days per week, one to three sets. If you are very ambitious and enjoy strength training, you may do it every day by alternating upper body one day and lower body the next. Keep a record of your accomplishments by marking the exercises done each day.

Exercise	Resistance	Repetitions	Sets
1. Bench press			
2. Overhead press			
3. Lateral pulls			
4. Lateral raises			
5. Bicep curls			
6. Squats			
7. Toe raises			
8. Abdominal curls			
9. Spine extensions			
10. Neck flexion			

Upper Body Workout	Resistance	Repetitions	Sets
1. Pec press			
2. Chest flys			
3. Biceps curl			
4. Lateral-side raises			
5. Triceps toner			
6. Chest press			

		Resistance	Repetitions	Sets
7.	Shoulder press			
8.	Triceps extension			
9.	One-arm row			
10.	Push-ups			

Lower Body Workout		*Resistance*	*Repetitions*	*Sets*
1.	Basic stomach crunch			
2.	Basic squats			
3.	Basic outer thigh leg lift			
4.	Basic inner thigh leg lift			
5.	Walking lunges			
6.	Calf raises			
7.	Oblique crunch			
8.	Buttocks firmer			
9.	Power lunge			